Mind Diet Cookbook For Seniors 2024

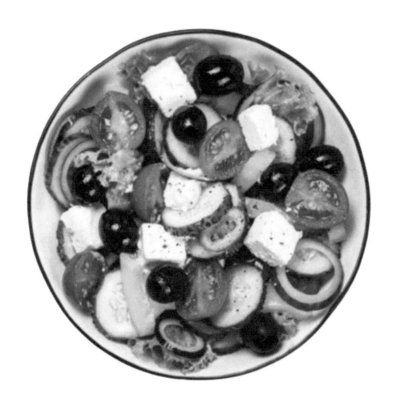

Discover Flavorful & Simple Meals for Your Healthy Transformation

Elva H. Miller

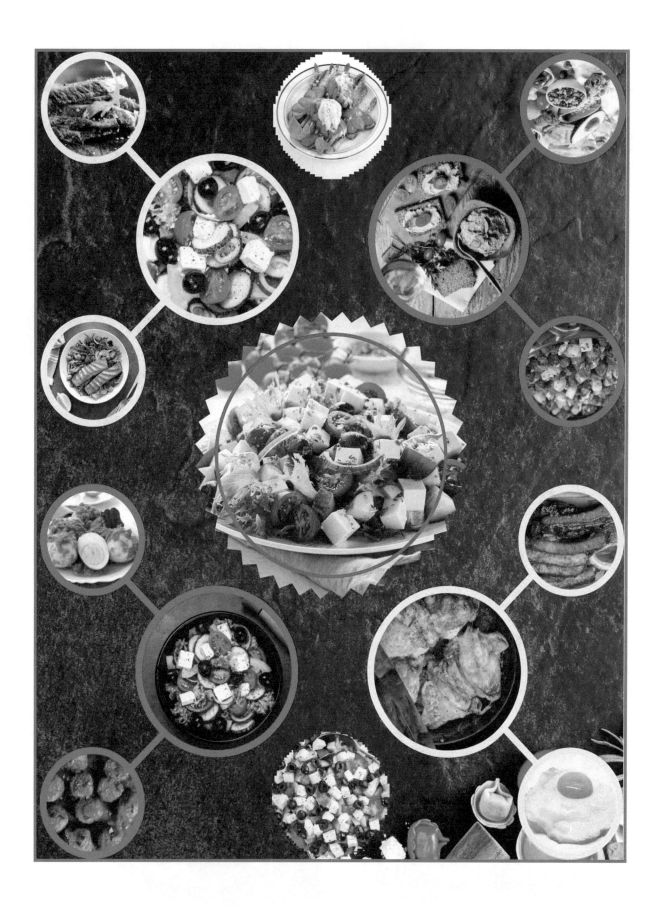

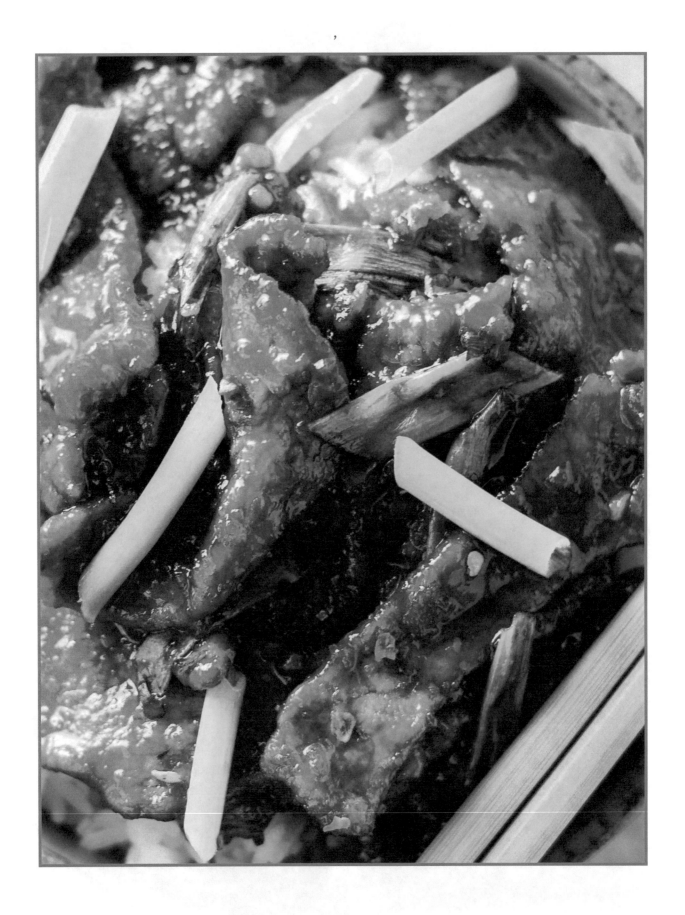

Contents

Introduction

Emma's Path to a Sharper Mind

Emma was always the glue that held her family together, noted for her quick wit and boundless enthusiasm. But as she entered her late sixties, she began to notice subtle changes. She occasionally misplaced her keys or struggled to recollect a familiar dish. These tiny lapses began to concern her. She believed they were early indicators of cognitive decline, a condition that had affected far too many of her friends.

Determined not to become another statistic, Emma started looking for ways to keep her mind sharp. She came across various publications and research that emphasized the role of food in cognitive performance. She discovered that some diets can improve brain function and memory. Emma, eager yet overwhelmed, realized she had no idea how to incorporate these brain-boosting nutrients into her everyday diet.

One afternoon, while exploring a local bookshop, Emma came upon a book that appeared to contain the answers she was looking for: **"Mind Diet Cookbook For Seniors 2024."** She immediately grabbed it up and began flicking through its pages. The book included delectable recipes, practical guidance, and straightforward instructions for promoting senior brain health.

Emma decided to try it. She began with a simple morning recipe: a berry smoothie loaded with antioxidants. The book walked her through each step, describing the benefits of each ingredient. She felt empowered because she was taking proactive actions to improve her memory and cognitive function.

Emma's kitchen changed throughout the course of several weeks. She experimented with new recipes such as quinoa and kale salad and baked salmon with walnut crust. The guidebook not only provided her with nutritional meals, but it also revived her desire to cook. Every successful dish she created increased her confidence.

Emma was not the only one who benefited from her newly acquired cooking skills. Her family was quick to note the shift. They were impressed with the variety and flavor of the dishes she prepared. Her granddaughters adored the berry and oat crisps she made for dessert, while her husband devoured the roasted vegetable and chickpea stew.

Emma felt a strong sense of accomplishment one evening as they sat around the dinner table, eating a substantial lentil and vegetable soup. She had taken control of her health and, as a result, brought her family closer together by preparing nutritious, tasty meals. The cookbook had given her more than just recipes; it had given her hope and a new sense of direction.

Emma's story spread to her friends and neighborhood. People were inspired by her makeover and wanted to learn her secret. She enthusiastically told her journey and recommended the **"Mind Diet Cookbook For Seniors 2024"** to anybody who listened.

"It's more than just a cookbook," she would explain. "It's a map toward a better life. It's about taking control of your health and enjoying each step along the way."

Emma's path demonstrates the value of the correct tools and expertise. With the "Mind Diet Cookbook For Seniors 2024," she transformed her anxiety and doubt into action and empowerment. If you want to improve your brain health while eating great, nutritious meals, this cookbook is the ideal companion.

Join Emma and millions of others who have discovered the advantages of the MIND diet. Invest in your health, enjoy every bite, and take the first step toward a brighter, healthier future with the **"Mind Diet Cookbook for Seniors 2024."** Your mind and body will appreciate you.

Welcome To The Book "Mind Diet Cookbook For Seniors 2024"

Your complete guide to improving brain health with delicious and nutritious meals. This book is intended to help elders achieve higher cognitive function, memory retention, and overall well-being. Whether you're experiencing early signs of cognitive decline or just want to keep your mind bright, this cookbook contains useful information and practical recipes to help you achieve your goals.

What This Book Is About

This cookbook is more than just a collection of dishes; it represents a holistic approach to brain health. We look at the science behind the MIND diet, a strong combo of the Mediterranean and DASH diets that has been shown to lower the risk of Alzheimer's disease and other types of dementia. You'll find extensive explanations of how different foods and nutrients promote brain health, as well as advice on meal planning, portion control, and efficient kitchen organization.

Who Can This Book Help?

This book is for seniors who desire to take proactive measures to improve their cognitive health. It's ideal for:

- ❖ **Individuals with mild cognitive impairments:** If you've seen changes in your memory or cognitive function, this book contains suggestions for potentially delaying these processes.
- ❖ **Caregivers and Family Members:** Caregivers of elderly loved ones will find useful tips for making brain-healthy meals that the entire family may enjoy.

- ❖ **Seniors Who Care About Their Health:** If you want to keep your cognitive abilities and overall health, this book will show you how to eat a well-balanced, healthy diet.

How This Book Will Help You

The **"Mind Diet Cookbook for Seniors 2024"** will provide you with the knowledge and skills to:

- ❖ **Boost Cognitive performance:** Discover how to include brain-boosting foods in your diet to improve memory, focus, and overall cognitive performance.
- ❖ **Enjoy Delicious Meals:** Discover a selection of delicious meals that enhance brain health while also being pleasurable and rewarding.
- ❖ **Simplify Meal Preparation:** Learn practical ideas for meal planning, grocery shopping, and cooking skills that can help you stick to a brain-healthy diet easily.
- ❖ **Stay Motivated:** With stories like Emma's path to greater brain health, you'll discover the inspiration and support you need to make long-term dietary changes.

A letter From The Author

My intention in making this cookbook is to have a good impact on the lives of elders everywhere. I want to demystify the concept of eating for brain health and demonstrate that it is not only possible, but also pleasant. Through this book, I intend to:

Educate: Provide clear, science-backed information on how nutrition affects brain health that is easily accessible and understanding.

Empower: Provide practical tools and great recipes to make the MIND diet a natural part of your daily routine.

Inspire: Share personal success stories and motivational suggestions to urge you to take charge of your health and enjoy the journey to improved brain function.

Join me on this journey towards a healthy mind and body. Let 2024 be the year we put brain health first and receive the delicious, nutritious advantages of the MIND diet. Your future self will thank you for investing in your health.

Welcome to a Healthier, Happier You with the **"Mind Diet Cookbook for Seniors 2024."** Let us go on this trip together!

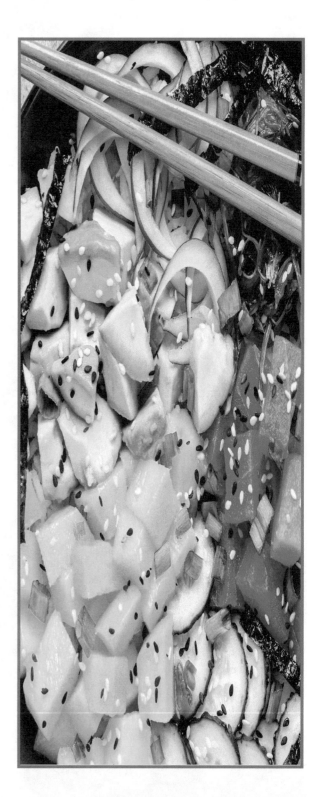

Chapter 1

The MIND diet

The Important of Brain Health for Seniors

As we get older, it becomes more important to preserve our brain health. Cognitive talents, such as memory, focus, and problem-solving ability, can deteriorate over time, lowering overall quality of life. Seniors should prioritize brain health for numerous important reasons:

- ❖ **Maintaining Independence:** Cognitive impairment can considerably impair daily tasks. Preserving brain health allows seniors to be more independent for longer, allowing them to manage personal affairs, negotiate social interactions, and pursue hobbies without requiring additional assistance.

- ❖ **Improving Quality of Life:** A sharp mind leads to a more satisfying life. Seniors with high cognitive function can continue to learn new things, have intriguing conversations, and participate in enjoyable and gratifying activities. This mental involvement promotes a sense of purpose and wellbeing.

- ❖ **Preventing Dementia:** Alzheimer's disease and other forms of dementia are serious problems for seniors. While there is no foolproof strategy to avoid these disorders, having a healthy brain can lower the chance or delay the onset of symptoms. A healthy diet, frequent physical activity, mental exercises, and social involvement are all beneficial to brain health.

- ❖ **Improving Emotional Well-Being:** Cognitive health is inextricably related to emotional health. Seniors with strong cognitive function tend to have better emotional stability and are less prone to suffer from despair and anxiety. A healthy brain enables elders to cope with the challenges and changes that come with age.

- ❖ **Social Engagement:** Maintaining cognitive abilities allows elders to stay in touch with family, friends, and the community. Social connections are important for emotional health and can improve cognitive function, resulting in a positive feedback loop that promotes general well-being.

❖ **Reducing Healthcare Costs:** Cognitive decline can result in higher healthcare needs, such as drugs, therapies, and long-term care. By focusing on brain health, seniors may be able to lower these costs, easing the financial strain on themselves and their families.

Tips for Maintaining Brain Health

A balanced diet with antioxidants, healthy fats, vitamins, and minerals promotes brain function. The MIND diet, which focuses on foods like leafy greens, berries, nuts, and whole grains, is especially beneficial.

❖ **Physical Activity:** Regular exercise boosts blood flow to the brain and promotes the formation of new brain cells. Walking, swimming, and yoga are great choices.

❖ **Mental Stimulation:** Doing cognitively demanding tasks like puzzles, reading, and learning new skills keeps the brain busy and sharp.

❖ **Social Connections:** Maintaining relationships and engaging in social activities can help to prevent cognitive deterioration.

❖ **Sleep:** Adequate sleep is essential for brain health since it promotes memory consolidation and cognitive function.

❖ **Stress Management:** Chronic stress can have a negative impact on brain health. Meditation, deep breathing exercises, and hobbies can all help you manage your stress.

How the MIND Diet Enhances Cognitive Function

The MIND diet, which stands for Mediterranean-DASH Diet Intervention for Neurodegenerative Delay, aims to improve brain health and lower the risk of cognitive decline. The MIND diet combines features of the Mediterranean and DASH diets, emphasizing nutrient-dense meals that promote cognitive performance and overall brain health. Here's how the MIND diet accomplishes these objectives:

❖ **Antioxidants:** These are essential for protecting brain cells from oxidative damage and inflammation, which can result in cognitive deterioration. The MIND diet promotes the consumption of antioxidant-rich fruits and vegetables, particularly berries and leafy greens, in order to neutralize free radicals and reduce inflammation, therefore safeguarding brain health.

❖ **High in Healthy Fats:** Healthy fats, particularly omega-3 fatty acids, are essential for brain building and function. The MIND diet includes omega-3-rich fish such as salmon, mackerel, and sardines. These lipids help develop and maintain cell membranes in the brain, enable communication between brain cells, and are linked to a lower risk of Alzheimer's disease.

❖ **Emphasis on Whole Grains:** Whole grains provide a consistent source of energy for the brain, helping it work throughout the day. Fiber-rich foods such as oats, quinoa, brown rice, and whole wheat aid to regulate blood sugar levels. Consistent energy supply is required for proper brain function, and whole grains include critical nutrients such as B vitamins, which are good for brain health.

❖ **Nuts and seeds** include a variety of nutrients that assist brain function, such as healthy fats, protein, fiber, vitamins and minerals. For example, almonds and walnuts, as well as flaxseed and chia seeds, contain vitamin E, which has been associated with a lower risk of cognitive decline. Regular eating of nuts and seeds as part of the MIND diet can improve cognitive performance and protect against neurodegenerative disease.

❖ **Low in Saturated Fats and Sugars:** The MIND diet restricts the consumption of saturated fats and sugars, which are linked to inflammation and an increased risk of cognitive impairment. Foods high in saturated fat, such as red meat and butter, are reduced, while sweets and processed foods are avoided. By minimizing these detrimental components, the MIND diet promotes healthy weight management, cardiovascular health, and lowers the risk of brain-impairing illnesses including diabetes and hypertension.

❖ **Moderate Wine Consumption:** The MIND diet emphasizes moderate wine consumption, particularly red wine. Red wine includes resveratrol, an antioxidant that may preserve the brain and improve cognitive function. However, wine should be consumed in moderation, as too much alcohol can have the reverse effect and impede brain function.

❖ **Supports Overall Cardiovascular Health:** Good cardiovascular health is intimately related to brain health. The MIND diet emphasizes heart-healthy foods such as whole grains, fatty salmon, nuts, and olive oil, which support healthy blood vessels and enough blood flow to the brain. Proper blood flow is critical for providing oxygen and nutrients to brain cells, hence supporting cognitive activities and overall brain health.

❖ **Promotes Balanced Meals and Consistent Eating Patterns:** The MIND diet promotes balanced meals with a range of nutrient-dense foods, ensuring that the brain obtains enough critical nutrients throughout the day. Consistent eating patterns help keep blood sugar levels consistent, preventing energy dips

and spikes that can impair cognitive performance.

Overview of the MIND Diet Principles

The MIND diet, or Mediterranean-DASH Diet Intervention for Neurodegenerative Delay, attempts to improve brain health and lower the risk of cognitive decline, including Alzheimer's disease. It combines features of the Mediterranean and DASH (Dietary Approaches to Stop Hypertension) diets, focusing on nutrient-dense meals that boost overall brain function. Here's an overview of the primary components of the MIND diet:

Focus on plant-based foods:

❖ **Leafy Green Vegetables:** Eat at least six servings of leafy green vegetables every week, including spinach, kale, and Swiss chard. These vegetables are high in vitamins, minerals, and antioxidants, which can help protect brain cells from injury.

❖ **Other veggies:** Eat at least one serving of other veggies per day. Choose a variety of bright veggies to acquire a diverse range of nutrients and antioxidants.

- ❖ **Berries:** Eat berries at least twice a week, preferably blueberries and strawberries. Berries include antioxidants and phytochemicals that improve brain health and cognitive performance.
- ❖ **Nuts:** Eat five servings of nuts each week. Nuts include healthful fats, vitamin E, and other elements that promote cognitive performance and prevent inflammation.

Inclusion of Healthy Fats:

- ❖ **Use olive oil as the primary cooking oil.** Olive oil contains monounsaturated fats and antioxidants, which protect brain cells and improve cardiovascular health.
- ❖ **Fish:** Consume fish at least once each week, ideally fatty fish such as salmon, mackerel, and sardines. Fish contains omega-3 fatty acids, which are necessary for proper brain construction and function.

Whole grains and legumes:

- ❖ **Whole Grains:** Eat at least three servings of whole grains each day, including oats, quinoa, brown rice, and whole wheat products. Whole grains contain fiber, B vitamins, and sustained energy, all of which are beneficial to cognitive performance and blood sugar stability.
- ❖ **Consume beans, lentils,** and other legumes at least four times per week. Legumes are high in plant-based protein, fiber, and minerals, which aid in brain function.

Moderate consumption of animal products

- ❖ **Poultry:** Eat poultry, such as chicken or turkey, at least twice per week. Poultry delivers lean protein and important elements while containing less saturated fat than red meat.
- ❖ **Red Meat:** Limit your red meat consumption to three servings per week. Red meat has been related to inflammation and cognitive impairment due to its high saturated fat content.
- ❖ **Limit high-fat dairy products.** Choose low-fat or fat-free dairy products to lower your saturated fat intake.

Limiting unhealthy foods:

- ❖ **Sweets and Pastries:** Limit your intake of sweets, pastries, and other foods high in added sugars and bad fats. These foods may cause inflammation and raise the risk of cognitive impairment.

- ❖ **Limit butter and margarine** to no more than one tablespoon every day. Choose healthier fats such as olive oil or avocado instead.

- ❖ **Reduce your intake of fried and fast foods,** which are heavy in harmful fats, sodium, and additives that might impair cognitive performance.

Moderate Wine Consumption:

- ❖ **Red Wine:** If you consume alcohol, have a glass of red wine every day. Red wine includes resveratrol, which is an antioxidant that may benefit the brain. However, moderation is crucial, as excessive alcohol use can impair brain function.

The MIND diet is a flexible and sustainable eating regimen that promotes brain function. The MIND diet, which emphasizes plant-based foods, healthy fats, whole grains, and lean proteins while restricting bad fats, sweets, and processed foods, offers a comprehensive framework for improving cognitive function and lowering the risk of neurodegenerative illnesses.

Adopting the MIND diet's principles can help seniors maintain mental sharpness, increase their quality of life, and reap the benefits of a nutritious, balanced diet.

Prioritizing brain health is critical for seniors to maintain independence, improve their quality of life, and lower healthcare expenses. The MIND diet, which focuses on nutrient-dense foods and healthy eating habits, is a scientifically sound approach to improving cognitive performance and overall well-being.

Seniors who follow the principles given in this guide can take proactive actions to maintain their brain health and live a meaningful, vibrant life.

Chapter 2
Getting Started

Essential Kitchen Tools and Equipment

To successfully follow the MIND diet, you must have the necessary tools and equipment in your kitchen. These items will assist you in cooking nutritious meals efficiently, allowing you to conveniently enjoy a variety of brain-boosting foods. Here's a list of essential kitchen tools and equipment to help you get started:

Cutting and Preparation Tools:

1. A high-quality chef's knife is required for cutting, slicing, and chopping fruits, vegetables, and other ingredients. A well-balanced, sharp knife makes food preparation safer and more efficient.

2. Paring Knife: This small knife is perfect for peeling and more complex tasks like chopping and coring fruits and vegetables.

3. To avoid cross-contamination, use separate cutting boards for vegetables, fruits, and meats. Choose durable materials like bamboo or polycarbonate.

4. Vegetable peeler: A robust vegetable peeler is essential to peel fruits and vegetables quickly and securely.

5. Kitchen shears are excellent for snipping herbs, cutting chicken, and doing other precise culinary tasks.

Mixing and Measuring Tools:

1. Mixing bowls: A collection of mixing bowls of various sizes is useful for blending materials, preparing salads, and creating dough. Bowls constructed of stainless steel or glass are durable and easy to clean.

2. Measuring cup and spoon: Accurate measuring tools are necessary for the following recipes. A set of measuring cups and spoons ensures precise measurements for both dry and liquid materials.

3. Food scales: A food scale is useful for measuring materials by weight, which is more accurate than volume measurements, especially for baking.

Cooking Tools:

1. Pots and pans: Buy multiple pots and pans, including a large stockpot, a medium-sized saucepan, a small saucepan, a nonstick skillet, and an iron skillet. These will meet the majority of your culinary needs.

2. Nonstick baking sheets and pans are essential for roasting vegetables, baking seafood, and preparing healthy snacks.

3. Steam Basket: A steamer basket allows you to steam vegetables while keeping their nutrients and vibrant colors.

4. A colander is used for draining pasta, rinsing beans, and cleaning fruits and vegetables.

5. Cooking Utensils: Stock your kitchen with a variety of cooking equipment, including wooden spoons, spatulas, tongs, ladles, and slotted spoons. These tools are necessary for stirring, flipping, and serving food.

6. Blender/Food Processor: A high-quality blender or food processor is required to make smoothies, purée soups, and create sauces and dips.

Storage and Organization:

1. Food Storage Containers: Have a few sealed containers on hand to keep leftovers, meal preps, and portioned snacks. Glass containers are durable and environmentally beneficial.

2. Mason jars: These containers are ideal for storing dry ingredients, making overnight oats, and serving salads and smoothies.

3. Spice Racks: Keep your spices fresh and accessible by storing them on a designated spice rack. Spices are essential for seasoning and delivering nutritional value to your food.

Specialty Tools:

1. A salad spinner is great for washing and drying leafy greens, ensuring they are crisp and ready to eat.

2. Microplane Grater: Finely grate citrus zest, garlic, ginger, and hard cheeses to improve the flavor of your meals.

3. Instant Pot or Slow Cooker: These appliances are perfect for preparing soups, stews, and whole grains with no effort. Slow cooking saves time and enhances flavor.

Beverage preparation:

1. An electric kettle quickly heats water for tea, oatmeal, and other hot beverages.

2. Coffee Makers: A dependable coffee maker ensures that you may enjoy your daily cup of coffee or tea, which can be a healthy element of a balanced diet when consumed moderately.

Having the right kitchen tools and equipment helps you cook nutritious, brain-healthy meals. Investing in these tools can make cooking more enjoyable and efficient, allowing you to stick to the MIND diet while reaping the cognitive benefits. Whether you're an experienced cook or just starting out, these tools may help you prepare delicious, nutritional meals that will boost your overall health and well-being.

Stock Your Pantry with MIND Diet Essentials

Creating a well-stocked pantry is a critical step in successfully implementing the MIND diet. Having the right ingredients on hand makes it easier to prepare healthy, brain-boosting meals and snacks. Here's how to stock your pantry with MIND diet basics.

Whole Grains:

- ❖ Oats are used to make oatmeal, granola, and baked products. They contain fiber and help keep blood sugar levels stable.
- ❖ Quinoa: This versatile grain can be used in salads, as a side dish, or instead of rice. Quinoa is high in protein and includes essential amino acids.
- ❖ Brown rice is a versatile whole grain with fiber, vitamins, and minerals.
- ❖ Whole Wheat Products: Keep whole wheat pasta, bread, and flour in your pantry to make nutritious meals and baked goods.
- ❖ Barley is a fiber-rich grain that works well in soups, stews, and salads. It also improves digestion and cardiovascular health.

Nuts and Seeds:

❖ Almonds are a delightful snack on their own or in salads, oatmeal, and baked goods. Almonds include healthy fats, vitamin E, and protein.

❖ Walnuts: High in omega-3 fatty acids, walnuts can be used in salads, baked items, or as snacks.

❖ Chia Seeds: Chia seeds can be used in smoothies, yogurt, and baked products to increase fiber, omega-3s, and protein content.

❖ Ground flaxseeds are a great source of omega-3s and fiber, and they may be used in smoothies, cereal, and baked goods.

❖ Pumpkin Seeds: Pumpkin seeds are a nutritious snack that may be added to salads and baked products. They are rich in antioxidants and healthy fats.

Legumes:

❖ Lentils: Save a variety of lentils (brown, green, and red) to use in soups, stews, and salads. Lentils are high in protein, fiber, and essential minerals.

❖ Black beans are abundant in protein, fiber, and antioxidants, so they make a great addition to salads, soups, and sides.

❖ Chickpeas are versatile and can be used in salads, stews, and hummus. They are a great source of protein and fiber.

❖ Kidney beans are high in protein and fiber, making them a great addition to chili, salads, and soup.

Healthy fats.

❖ Extra virgin olive oil includes monounsaturated fats and antioxidants, making it an essential ingredient in cooking, sauces, and marinades.

❖ Avocado Oil: A good substitute for olive oil with a high smoke point, suitable for cooking and baking.

❖ Nut Butters: Have almond and peanut butter on hand for snacking, smoothies, and baked items. Choose natural ones that contain no added sugars or hydrogenated fats.

Spices and herbs:

❖ Turmeric: Turmeric, recognized for its anti-inflammatory properties, is useful in cooking and baking.

- Cinnamon: It adds flavor to oatmeal, smoothies, and baked goods while also delivering antioxidant benefits.
- Garlic powder is a versatile spice that adds taste to many dishes while also delivering health benefits.
- Dry Herbs: Keep a variety of dried herbs on hand, including basil, oregano, thyme, and rosemary, to add flavor and nutrition to your meals.

Canned and jarred foods:

- Soups, stews, and pasta all require canned or jarred tomatoes as well as tomato sauce.
- Olives are a good source of healthy fats and antioxidants, and they may be used in salads, pasta meals, and as snacks.
- Artichoke hearts add texture and flavor to salads, pastas, and pizzas, plus they are strong in antioxidants.

Additional Essentials:

- Apple cider vinegar is useful in dressings and marinades and may have health benefits such as improved digestion and blood sugar management.
- Honey: Honey, a natural sweetener used in tea, yogurt, and baking, is also high in antioxidants.
- Low-sodium broth: Have vegetable, chicken, or beef broth on hand for soups, stews, and cereals.

Fresh produce:

- Berries: Fresh or frozen blueberries, strawberries, and raspberries can be utilized in smoothies, oatmeal, and snacks.
- Leafy greens: Keep fresh spinach, kale, and other greens on hand for salads, smoothies, and recipes.
- Cruciferous vegetables: Include broccoli, cauliflower, and Brussels sprouts in your regular grocery list for brain-boosting nutrients.

Stocking your cupboard with MIND diet basics ensures that you have all you need to prepare tasty, brain-healthy meals. By keeping these requirements on hand, you may simply follow the MIND diet principles and improve cognitive function and overall well-being. Whether you're making something from scratch or looking for a quick and healthful snack, these pantry basics lay the framework for a brain-boosting diet.

Meal Planning and Preparation Tips

To successfully follow the MIND diet, you must not only choose the right foods, but also plan and prepare them correctly. Here are some practical meal planning and preparation ideas to help you stay on track and include healthy eating into your daily routine.

1. Prepare a weekly meal plan.

Plan your meals.

- ❖ Make time each week to plan your meals, including breakfast, lunch, dinner, and snacks.
- ❖ Choose meals that contain MIND diet essentials like leafy greens, berries, almonds, whole grains, and healthy fats.

Balance Your Diet:

- ❖ Make sure your meal plan includes a variety of meals to provide a wide range of nutrients.

- ❖ Include a range of protein sources, such as fish, lentils, and lean poultry, as well as plenty of vegetables and whole grains.

2. Create a shopping list.

Organize by Category:

- ❖ To make grocery shopping easier, make a list based on your meal plan and categorize items (fruit, cereals, meats, etc.).

Stick with the list:

- ❖ Stick to your list to minimize impulse purchases and make sure you only buy materials for your planned meals.

Buy in quantity.

- ❖ Purchase basic commodities in bulk, such as cereals, nuts, and canned products, to save money and ensure that you always have the required supplies on hand.

3. Prepare the ingredients ahead of time.

Wash and cut vegetables:

❖ Wash, peel, and cut vegetables ahead of time, then place them in airtight containers in the refrigerator. This makes it simple to grab and use them for dinners throughout the week.

Cook Grains in Advance:

❖ Cook large quantities of healthful grains like quinoa, brown rice, and barley and store them in the fridge or freezer. These can be quickly incorporated into meals as needed.

Prepare proteins.

Pre-cook proteins such as chicken breasts, beans, and lentils. Store them in the refrigerator for easy usage in salads, wraps, and other dishes.

4. Batch cooking and freezing.

Batch Cooked Meals:

❖ Prepare a large batch of soups, stews, and casseroles and divide them into individual servings. Freeze these meals for quick, healthy options on busy days.

Label and Date:

❖ Label and date any prepared and cooked items stored in the refrigerator or freezer to maintain freshness and avoid waste.

5. Smart storage solutions.

Use clear containers.

❖ Store prepared ingredients and leftovers in clear containers so you can see what you've got.

Vacuum Seal:

❖ Purchase a vacuum sealer to extend the shelf life of fresh produce, meats, and pre-cooked meals stored in your freezer.

Organize the refrigerator:

❖ To make dinner preparation quicker and faster, combine similar items and store them in separate refrigerator compartments.

6. Simplify the cooking procedure.

One-Pan Meals:

❖ Choose one-pan or one-pot meals to reduce cleanup and simplify cooking. Roasted vegetables and sheet pan dishes are great options.

Use kitchen gadgets.

❖ Slow cookers, pressure cookers, and blenders can help you save time in the kitchen when preparing meals.

Embrace no-cook recipes.

❖ Include no-cook recipes like salads and overnight oats in your meal plan for quick and nutritious dinners.

7. Keep nutritious snacks handy.

Prepare Snacks Ahead:

❖ Prepare healthful snacks like almonds, cut-up fruits, and vegetable

sticks early in the week so they're ready to go when needed.

Create Snack Packs:

❖ Create snack packs including protein, healthy fats, and fiber to keep you filled between meals.

8. Maintain flexibility and adaptability.

Adjust for availability:

❖ Adjust your meal plan to reflect seasonal vegetables and what is on sale at the grocery store.

Incorporate leftovers.

❖ Plan for leftovers by including meals that can be easily transformed into other dishes. For example, mix leftover roasted vegetables into a salad or wrap.

Listen to your body.

❖ Be conscious of your hunger and fullness cues, and adjust portion sizes and meal time to meet your specific needs.

9. Involve Family and Friends

Cook together.

❖ Involve your family and friends in meal preparation. This may make cooking more enjoyable and less stressful.

Share meals.

❖ Sharing meals with friends or neighbors can offer variety while saving time on meal preparation.

Effective meal planning and preparation are essential for following the MIND diet and reaping its cognitive benefits. Healthy eating may be made more convenient and enjoyable by planning your meals, prepping foods ahead of time, and utilizing clever storage options. These suggestions will help you keep to the MIND diet by ensuring that you consume nutrient-dense, brain-boosting meals on a regular basis.

Understanding Serving Sizes and Portions.

Proper portion control is essential for eating a balanced meal and obtaining adequate nutrients without overeating. Understanding portion sizes and quantities allows you to manage your consumption of various meals, which is critical while following the MIND diet. Here's a tool to help you better comprehend serving sizes and quantities:

1. What is the serving size?

❖ ***Definition:*** A serving size is a set amount of food recommended by dietary guidelines. It is commonly used on nutrition labels to indicate how much of a nutrient you are receiving.

❖ ***Guidelines:*** Health authorities, such as the FDA, set serving sizes and use them as a benchmark to ensure you get the right nutritional balance.

2. Common Serving Sizes:

❖ ***Vegetables:*** A serving of vegetables typically includes one cup of raw leafy greens and half a cup of cooked or raw non-leafy vegetables.

❖ ***Fruit*** servings typically consist of one medium fruit (such as an apple or banana), half a cup of fresh, frozen, or canned fruit, or a quarter cup of dried fruit.

- ❖ *A serving of whole grains* is one slice of whole grain bread, half a cup of cooked grains (such as brown rice or quinoa), or one ounce of dry cereal.
- ❖ *Nuts and seeds:* A normal portion of nuts or seeds is one ounce, which is equivalent to a small handful or two teaspoons.
- ❖ *Legumes:* One serving is half a cup of cooked legumes like beans or lentils.
- ❖ *Fish:* A serving of fish typically weighs three to four ounces, which is about the size of a deck of cards.
- ❖ *Poultry and meat:* A serving of chicken or meat is usually three ounces, which is roughly the size of a deck of cards.
- ❖ *Dairy:* One serving equals one cup of milk or yogurt, or one and a half ounces of cheese.
- ❖ *Healthy fats:* One tablespoon of healthy fat, such as olive oil, equals one serving.

3. Tips for Estimating Portion Size.

- ❖ *Use your hand:* Your hand could be a useful tool for estimating portion sizes. For example, a fist is about the size of a cup, a palm is around the size of a three-ounce meal of meat, and a thumb is about the size of one tablespoon of fat.
- ❖ *Visual cues:* Use familiar objects to estimate portion size. A deck of cards is equivalent to one serving of meat, a tennis ball to one cup of fruits or vegetables, and a golf ball to 1/4 cup of nuts or seeds.
- ❖ *Measuring tools:* To accurately measure amounts, utilize measuring cups, spoons, and a food scale, especially if you are unfamiliar with standard serving sizes.

4. Portion Control Strategies.

- ❖ *Pre-portion Snacks:* To avoid overeating, divide items into individual servings ahead of time. Compact containers or snack bags are ideal for storing individual portions of nuts, fruits, and vegetables.
- ❖ *Instead of placing* serving dishes on the table, serve meals directly to plates from the kitchen. This allows you to control your serving sizes and avoid the temptation to go for seconds.

- ❖ **Use tiny plates and bowls:** Smaller dishes can make servings appear larger, making you feel fuller with less food.

- ❖ **Eat slowly and mindfully:** Take your time with your meals, chew thoroughly, and enjoy every bite. This allows your brain to identify fullness, which reduces overeating.

- ❖ **Fill Half Your Plate With Vegetables:** Aim to fill half of your plate with vegetables, one-quarter with lean protein, and one-quarter with nutritious carbohydrates. This keeps the dish balanced and nutrient-dense.

- ❖ **Avoid eating straight** from the package: Instead of eating straight from the container, portion food onto a plate or bowl to avoid mindless munching and larger servings.

5. Reading Nutrition Labels.

- ❖ Check the serving size listed on the nutrition label to see how much food the nutritional information refers to.

- ❖ **Total servings per container:** Keep track of the total number of servings in each container to avoid accidentally eating too much in one sitting.

- ❖ **Nutrient content:** Use the nutrition label to track your calorie, fat, sugar, and nutrient intake, and adjust your portion sizes to meet your dietary goals.

Understanding serving sizes and quantities is crucial for maintaining a healthy diet and acquiring enough nutrients. You may enhance your overall health by becoming familiar with standard serving sizes, using portion control strategies, and paying attention to nutrition labels.

These activities are especially important while following the MIND diet because they allow you to maximize the cognitive benefits of the foods you eat while still eating a balanced and healthy diet.

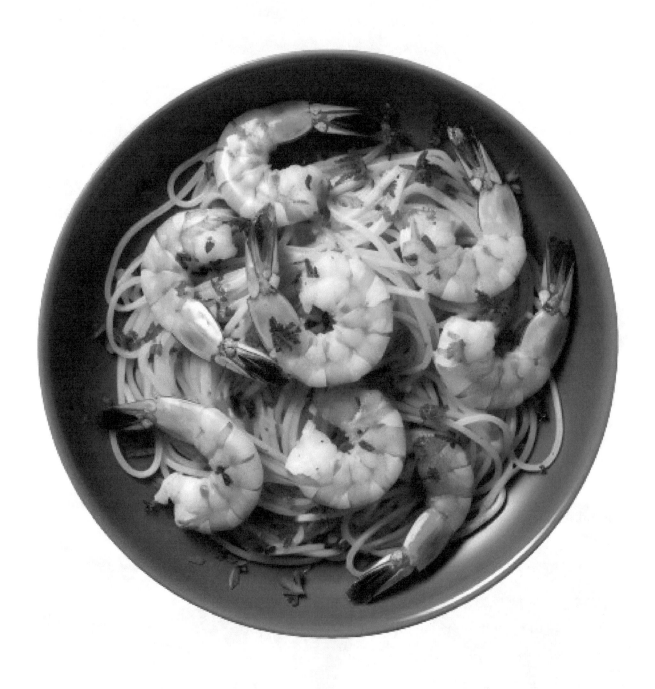

Chapter 3

Healthy and Delicious Recipes For Brain Health

Energizing Breakfasts Recipes

1. Vegetable-Packed Frittata

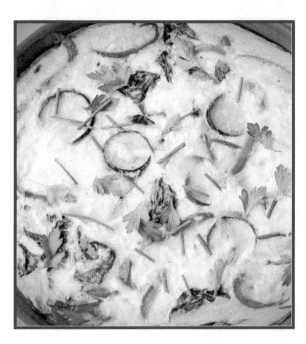

A frittata is a flexible and tasty Italian meal made with eggs, cheese, and veggies. This veggie-packed version is full of colorful flavor and makes an excellent breakfast, brunch, lunch, or supper.

- ❖ **Preparation time:** 10 minutes
- ❖ **Cook time:** 25 minutes
- ❖ **Total time:** 35 minutes

Ingredients:

- ❖ 8 big eggs.
- ❖ 1/2 cup milk, either dairy or non-dairy.
- ❖ 1 tablespoon of olive oil.
- ❖ 1 tiny, chopped onion
- ❖ 1 red bell pepper, chopped
- ❖ 1 cup of chopped broccoli florets.
- ❖ 1 cup of chopped spinach.
- ❖ 1/2 cup cherry tomatoes (halved)
- ❖ 1/2 cup of shredded cheddar cheese (or your favorite cheese).
- ❖ 1/2 teaspoon of dried oregano.
- ❖ Add salt and pepper to taste.

Instructions:

- ❖ Preheat the oven to 400 °F (200 °C). Grease a 10-inch ovenproof pan with olive oil.
- ❖ In a large mixing basin, whisk together the eggs and milk. Season with salt, pepper, and oregano.
- ❖ Heat olive oil in a pan over medium heat. Cook the onion and bell pepper

for approximately 5 minutes, or until softened.

- ❖ Add the broccoli and simmer for another 2-3 minutes, or until slightly tender-crisp.
- ❖ Add the spinach and simmer until wilted.
- ❖ Pour the egg mixture into the pan, then toss in the cooked veggies. Top with cherry tomatoes and cheddar cheese.
- ❖ Bake for 20-25 minutes, or until the eggs have set and the cheese is melted and bubbling.
- ❖ Allow the frittata to cool slightly before slicing and serving.

Serving size per recipe: 6 wedges.

Nutrition Information:

- ❖ Calories: Per serving (roughly one-sixth of the recipe), around 250 calories
- ❖ Carbohydrate: 10 grams
- ❖ Fat: 15g
- ❖ Protein: 15 grams.
- ❖ Vitamin A: An excellent source (from red bell pepper).
- ❖ Vitamin C: A good supply (from broccoli).

- ❖ Fiber: 2 grams.

Cooking Tips:

- ❖ Full-fat milk and cheese provide a fuller taste.
- ❖ You may make this dish with your favorite veggies. Other fantastic possibilities are zucchini, mushrooms, asparagus, and sun-dried tomatoes.
- ❖ If you don't have an ovenproof pan, cook a frittata on the stove top for a few minutes until the bottom is set before moving it to a preheated broiler to finish cooking the top.
- ❖ Leftovers can be refrigerated for up to three days. Reheat gently in a skillet or microwave.

Health Benefits:

- ❖ Frittatas have plenty of protein, which keeps you full and pleased.
- ❖ They also include vitamins and minerals from the veggies.
- ❖ This dish is an excellent way to start the day off right with a nutritious and tasty meal.

2. Whole-Grain Avocado Toast

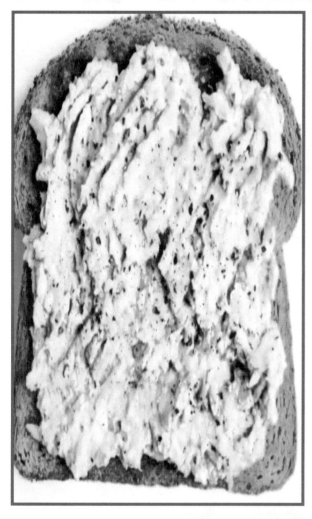

Whole grain avocado toast is a popular breakfast option, and for good reason. It's quick, simple to prepare, and high in healthy fats, fiber, and critical nutrients.

- ❖ **Preparation time:** 5 minutes
- ❖ **Cooking time**: 2-3 minutes (depending on the toaster).
- ❖ **Total time:** 7–8 minutes

Ingredients:

- ❖ 1 piece of whole-grain bread (such as wheat, rye, or Ezekiel bread).
- ❖ ½ ripe avocado.
- ❖ ½ lemon juice (optional)
- ❖ Pinch of salt.
- ❖ A pinch of black pepper.
- ❖ *Optional Toppings:* Sliced cherry tomatoes, crumbled feta cheese, everything bagel spice, chopped fresh herbs (such as cilantro or chives).

Instructions:

- ❖ Toast your bread to the desired crispness.
- ❖ While the bread is browning, halve the avocado, remove the pit, and scoop out the meat. In a bowl, mash the avocado with a fork until it reaches the desired consistency, which can be chunky or smooth.
- ❖ (Optional) If used, sprinkle the avocado with lemon juice to keep it from browning.
- ❖ Season the mashed avocado with salt and pepper to taste.
- ❖ Spread the mashed avocado on toasted bread.

- ❖ Top with your preferred toppings (optional).
- ❖ Each recipe yields one serving.

Nutrition Facts: (Per serving, based on usual components)

- ❖ Calories: 220
- ❖ Carbohydrate: 25 grams
- ❖ Fat: 10g
- ❖ Protein: 5 grams.
- ❖ Vitamin C: 2 milligrams (if lemon juice is used).
- ❖ Fiber: 5 grams.

Cooking Tips:

- ❖ To fully ripen an avocado, place it in a brown paper bag alongside an apple or banana for a day or two.
- ❖ If your avocado isn't quite ripe, toast the bread for a little longer to provide warmth and soften the avocado when spread.
- ❖ Drizzle the bread with olive oil before adding the mashed avocado for a more flavorful finish.

Health Benefits:

Whole grain avocado toast is a well-balanced breakfast option that may keep you full and content all morning. Here's a summary of some important health benefits:

- ❖ Avocados are high in monounsaturated fats, which can benefit heart health and enhance feelings of fullness.
- ❖ Fiber: Whole-grain bread and avocado both contain fiber, which is beneficial to digestion and intestinal health.
- ❖ Whole grains include critical vitamins and minerals, whereas avocado is high in vitamin C and potassium.
- ❖ Whole grain avocado toast is a breakfast choice that will keep you going all morning thanks to its simplicity, excellent flavor, and remarkable nutritional profile.

3. Avocado toast with tomato and basil

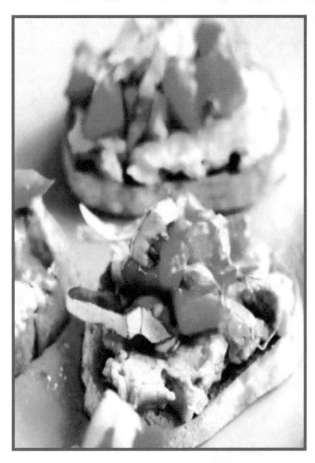

Avocado toast with tomato and basil is a traditional breakfast choice that is both tasty and nutritious. It's an excellent way to begin the day with a filling combination of healthy fats, fiber, and critical vitamins.

- ❖ **Preparation time:** 5 minutes
- ❖ **Cooking Time:** (Not relevant; toasting bread only)
- ❖ **Total time:** 5 minutes.

Ingredients:

- ❖ 1 piece of whole wheat bread.
- ❖ 1/2 ripe avocado.
- ❖ 1 small tomato, thinly sliced
- ❖ 1/4 cup fresh basil leaves, coarsely chopped
- ❖ 1 tablespoon of extra virgin olive oil.
- ❖ A pinch of sea salt.
- ❖ Add freshly ground black pepper to taste.

Instructions:

- ❖ Toast the bread to the desired crispness.
- ❖ While the bread is browning, halve the avocado, remove the pit, and scoop out the meat.
- ❖ Mash the avocado with a fork on a dish, leaving it somewhat chunky.
- ❖ Spread the mashed avocado evenly over the toasted bread.
- ❖ Top with sliced tomato and chopped basil.
- ❖ Drizzle with olive oil, season with salt and pepper as desired, and enjoy!

Serving size: Each recipe yields one serving.

Nutrition information:

- ❖ Calories: 280
- ❖ Carbs: 30g
- ❖ Fat: 15g
- ❖ Protein: 5 grams.
- ❖ Vitamin K: 25 percent DV
- ❖ Fiber: 7 grams.

Cooking Tips:

- ❖ Cooking For a more delicious avocado, add fresh lemon juice before mashing.
- ❖ If your tomatoes aren't particularly delicious, try dusting them with salt and sugar before toasting.
- ❖ To add protein, top your toast with crumbled feta cheese or a poached egg.
- ❖ Switch things up! This recipe makes an excellent base; feel free to experiment with other toppings such as a sprinkling of balsamic glaze, a dash of spicy sauce, or even a dollop of pesto.

Health Benefits:

- ❖ Avocado toast is an excellent method to include healthy fats to your diet. Avocados include monounsaturated fats, which can benefit heart health. They are also high in fiber, which can make you feel fuller and more pleased. Tomatoes are high in vitamins A and C, whereas basil contains antioxidants.

4. Quinoa porridge with Berries

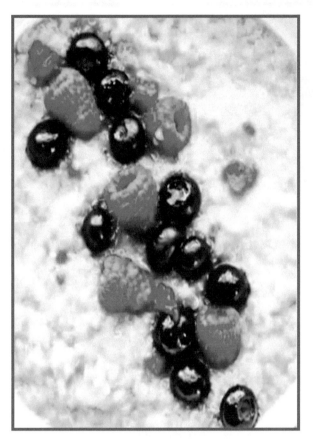

Quinoa porridge with berries is a tasty and nutritious breakfast alternative that's ideal for hectic mornings. The quinoa provides protein and fiber, while the berries offer flavor and antioxidants. This recipe may be readily modified with your own toppings and milk alternatives.

- ❖ **Preparation time:** 5 minutes
- ❖ **Cook time:** 15 minutes
- ❖ **Total time:** 20 minutes

Ingredients:

- ❖ ½ cup washed quinoa.
- ❖ 1 cup water.
- ❖ 1 ¾ cup milk, either dairy or non-dairy.
- ❖ ¼ teaspoon of ground cinnamon
- ❖ Pinch of salt.
- ❖ 1 cup fresh or frozen berries (such as strawberries, blueberries, and raspberries).
- ❖ 1 tablespoon maple syrup (or any sweetener of your preference)
- ❖ 1/4 cup chopped nuts and seeds (optional)
- ❖ 1/4 cup shredded coconut (optional)

Instructions:

- ❖ In a saucepan, mix the washed quinoa, water, milk, cinnamon, and salt. Bring to a boil over medium heat.
- ❖ Reduce the heat to low, cover the pan, and cook for 15 minutes, or until the quinoa is fully cooked and the liquid has been absorbed.
- ❖ Remove from heat and add the berries and maple syrup.
- ❖ Serve warm in bowls and sprinkle with your favorite chopped nuts,

seeds, and shredded coconut (optional).

Serving Size: One serving

Nutrition Facts: (per serving)

- ❖ Calories: 350.
- ❖ Carbohydrates: 50g, 5g fat, 8g protein.
- ❖ Fiber: 5 grams.
- ❖ Vitamin C: 10 percent DV
- ❖ Manganese: 20 percent. DV

Cooking Tips:

- ❖ For a creamier porridge, use extra milk or finish with a dash of heavy cream.
- ❖ If the porridge becomes too thick after cooking, add a bit of extra water or milk.
- ❖ To save time in the morning, cook the quinoa the night before and refrigerate in an airtight container. Simply reheat with milk and fruit in the morning.

Health Benefits:

- ❖ Quinoa is a complete protein, which means it includes all nine important amino acids your body needs.
- ❖ It also contains fiber, which makes you feel full and content.
- ❖ Berries are rich in antioxidants, which can help protect your cells from harm.
- ❖ This morning porridge is an excellent way to start the day with a boost of energy and minerals.

5. Spinach and Feta Scramble.

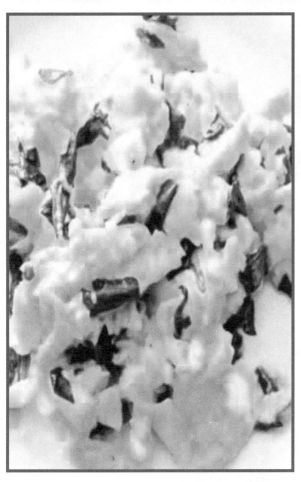

Spinach and Feta Scramble is a tasty and protein-packed breakfast option that takes less than 15 minutes to prepare. It's loaded with nutrients from the spinach and feta cheese, giving it a nutritious and filling way to start the day.

- ❖ **Preparation time:** 5 minutes
- ❖ **Cooking time:** 10 minutes
- ❖ **Total time:** 15 minutes

Ingredients:

- ❖ 2 huge eggs.
- ❖ 1 tablespoon of olive oil.
- ❖ 3 cups fresh spinach, coarsely chopped.
- ❖ 1/4 cup crumbled feta cheese.
- ❖ Add salt and black pepper to taste (optional). Add ¼ cup sliced cherry tomatoes (optional). ¼ teaspoon dried oregano.

Instructions:

- ❖ In a mixing dish, whisk together the eggs, salt, and pepper.
- ❖ In a medium-size pan, heat the olive oil. Cook the spinach, stirring periodically, until wilted (approximately 2 minutes).
- ❖ Push the spinach to the edge of the pan. Pour the egg mixture into the middle of the pan. Allow it to settle for a few seconds before gently folding the cooked sides into the middle. Continue folding the eggs until they are nearly set but still slightly moist.
- ❖ Remove from the heat and mix in the crumbled feta cheese. If using, combine the cherry tomatoes and

oregano. Season with more salt and pepper to taste.

Serving Size: One serving

Nutrition Facts: (Per Serving)

- ❖ Calories: 240
- ❖ Carbohydrates: 6g, Fat: 14g.
- ❖ Protein: 16 grams.
- ❖ Vitamin A: 20% of the Daily Value
- ❖ Vitamin C: 15 percent DV
- ❖ Iron: 10% DV
- ❖ Fiber: 2 grams.

Cooking Tips:

- ❖ For creamier eggs, add a spoonful of milk or cream cheese to the eggs.
- ❖ Do not overcook the eggs. They will continue to cook even after being removed from the fire.
- ❖ To prepare this meal ahead of time, scramble the eggs and sauté the spinach. Keep them separate in the refrigerator for up to two days. Reheat gently in a pan over low heat until heated through.

Health Benefits:

- ❖ Eggs are a high-protein food that keeps you full and content.
- ❖ Spinach is a leafy green vegetable rich in vitamins, minerals, and antioxidants.
- ❖ Feta cheese is a rich source of calcium and protein.
- ❖ This scramble is a low-carb, keto-friendly breakfast choice.

6. Mushroom & Spinach Scramble

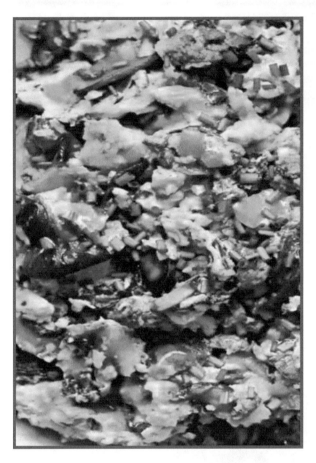

This quick and easy Mushroom and Spinach Scramble is an excellent way to begin the day. The eggs provide protein, the spinach provides vitamins and fiber, while the mushrooms add a delicious flavor. This recipe takes less than 15 minutes to prepare, making it excellent for hectic mornings.

- ❖ **Preparation time: 5** minutes
- ❖ **Cooking time:** 10 minutes
- ❖ **Total time:** 15 minutes

Ingredients:

- ❖ 1/2 tablespoon of olive oil.
- ❖ 1/4 cup minced onion
- ❖ 1/2 cup sliced mushrooms (cremini, white button, or your preferred kind)
- ❖ 1/2 cup of fresh baby spinach.
- ❖ 2 huge eggs.
- ❖ 1 big egg white (optional for added protein)
- ❖ 1 teaspoon water.
- ❖ Add kosher salt and freshly ground black pepper to taste.
- ❖ 2 tablespoons shredded cheese (gruyere, cheddar, or your favorite) (optional)

Instructions:

- ❖ In a small mixing bowl, combine the eggs, egg white (if using), water, a teaspoon of salt, and pepper.
- ❖ In a medium-sized nonstick skillet, heat the olive oil over medium heat. Cook the onions for 3-4 minutes, until they are softened and transparent.
- ❖ Cook the sliced mushrooms for a further 3-4 minutes, or until soft and slightly golden brown.

- Push the mushrooms and onions to the sides of the pan. Cook the spinach, turning occasionally, until wilted, approximately 1-2 minutes.
- Pour the egg mixture evenly into the pan. As the eggs begin to set, use a spatula to carefully bring cooked pieces to the center, allowing the runny egg to fill in the gaps. Continue cooking until the eggs are almost set, leaving some soft curds.
- If using cheese, add it to the scramble and heat for an additional minute, or until melted and gooey.
- Remove from the heat and serve immediately.

Serving Size: One serving

Nutrition Information:

- **Calories:** around 280 (depending on the kind and quantity of cheese used).
- **Carbohydrate:** 5 grams
- **Fat:** 15g
- **Protein:** 20 grams (with egg white)
- **Vitamin A:** excellent supply (from spinach).
- **Vitamin C:** Good source (from spinach).
- **Iron:** A good source (from spinach).
- **Fiber:** 2 grams.

Cooking Tips:

- To make creamier scrambled eggs, add a dash of milk or cream to the egg mixture.
- If you don't have fresh spinach, you may substitute frozen spinach. Before you put it in the pan, thaw it and wring out any extra liquid.
- Want to add additional vegetables? Try adding diced bell peppers, tomatoes, or broccoli to the scramble.
- Play with various cheeses! Feta, goat cheese, and Parmesan would all be excellent choices.

Health Benefits:

- This Mushroom and Spinach Scramble is a nutritional powerhouse. Eggs are an excellent source of complete protein, which keeps you full and happy. Spinach is high in vitamins and minerals, including A and C, iron, and fiber.

7. *Greek yogurt parfait with granola*

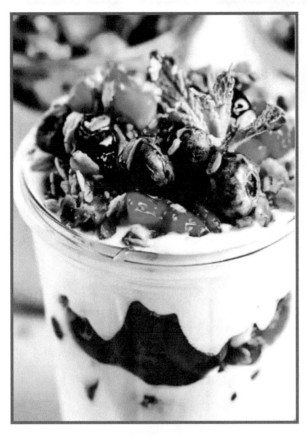

A nutritious and tasty parfait is an excellent way to start the day or as a delightful afternoon snack. This Greek Yogurt Parfait with Granola is packed with protein, fiber, and fresh fruit tastes, making it simple to personalize and meal prep for busy mornings.

- ❖ **Preparation time:** 5 minutes
- ❖ **Cooking time:** 0 minutes
- ❖ **Total time:** 5 minutes

Ingredients:

- ❖ 1 container (6 ounces) Plain Greek Yogurt
- ❖ 1/2 cup granola, homemade or store-bought.
- ❖ 1/2 cup fresh or frozen fruit (such as berries, mangos, and bananas).
- ❖ 1 tablespoon of honey or maple syrup (optional).
- ❖ 1/4 teaspoon vanilla extract (optional).

Instructions:

- ❖ In a mixing bowl, combine the Greek yogurt, honey or maple syrup, and vanilla extract (if using). Stir until well blended.
- ❖ Divide the yogurt mixture into two glasses or bowls.
- ❖ Top each plate with half the granola and half the fruit.
- ❖ Enjoy right now!

Serving size per recipe: 2 servings.

Nutritional Information:

- ❖ **Calories:** 300-400 calories.
- ❖ **Carbohydrate:** 30-40 grams.

- ❖ **Fat:** 5-10 g
- ❖ **Protein:** 20-30 g.
- ❖ **Vitamin A:** From Greek yogurt and berries.
- ❖ **Vitamin C:** comes from fruit.
- ❖ **Fiber:** comes from granola and fruit.

Cooking Tips:

- ❖ To make a thicker parfait, use thicker Greek yogurt or refrigerate the mixture for 30 minutes before assembling.
- ❖ To prepare this recipe ahead of time, place the parfaits in lidded mason jars and refrigerate for up to two days. To avoid soggy granola, keep it separate from the yogurt and fruit until ready to serve.

- ❖ Be creative with your toppings! Chopped nuts, chia seeds, shredded coconut, or a splash of nut butter are all tasty toppings.

Health Benefits:

- ❖ Greek yogurt contains a high concentration of protein, which keeps you full and happy.
- ❖ Granola contains fiber, which is beneficial for digestion and intestinal health.
- ❖ Fresh fruits are loaded with vitamins, minerals, and antioxidants.
- ❖ This parfait is a well-balanced supper or snack that may keep you energized all day.

Chapter 4

Brain-Boosting Snacks and Small Bites

1. Roasted chickpeas

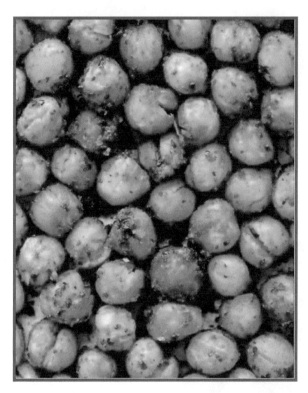

Roasted chickpeas are a nutritious, crispy snack that will fulfill your desires without relying on harmful chips or fries. They are a good source of plant-based protein and fiber, and they may be readily spiced to suit your tastes.

- ❖ **Preparation time:** 5 minutes
- ❖ **Cooking time:** 20-30 minutes
- ❖ **Total time:** 25-35 minutes

Ingredients:

- 1 (15-ounce) can of drained and washed chickpeas.
- 1 tablespoon of olive oil.
- 1/2 teaspoon of salt.
- 1/4 teaspoon black pepper (optional).
- Additional spices of your choosing (as suggested in Cooking Tips below)

Instructions:

- ❖ Preheat the oven to 425°F (220°C). Line a baking sheet with parchment paper for easy cleaning.
- ❖ Dry the chickpeas with a clean kitchen towel. The drier the chickpeas, the crispier they get.
- ❖ In a large bowl, combine the chickpeas, olive oil, salt, and black pepper (if using).
- ❖ Place the chickpeas in a single layer on the prepared baking sheet.
- ❖ Roast for 20-30 minutes, or until the chickpeas turn golden brown and

crispy. Shake the pan occasionally to achieve even frying.

❖ Toss in any additional spices while the chickpeas are still heated.

❖ Allow the chickpeas to cool slightly before serving.

Serving size: around 1/2 cup.

Nutrition Facts (per 1/2 cup serving)

- **Calories:** 160
- **Carbs:** 20 grams
- **Fat:** 5 g.
- **Protein:** 6 g.
- **Fiber:** 5 g
- **Vitamin C:** 2%. DV
- **Iron:** 10% DV

Cooking Tips:

❖ Remove the skins off the chickpeas before roasting to get them extra crispy. Simply rub the dry chickpeas between your thumb and forefinger.

❖ Experiment with various taste combinations! Here are a few ideas:

  ➢ **Savory:** Garlic powder, onion powder, smoked paprika, cumin, chili powder, curry powder, and Italian seasoning.

  ➢ **Spicy:** Cayenne pepper, red pepper flakes, and sriracha

  ➢ **Sweet:** cinnamon, nutmeg, maple syrup, brown sugar (use sparingly).

❖ Allow the roasted chickpeas to completely cool before storing in an airtight jar at room temperature. They will remain crisp for up to three days.

Health Benefits:

❖ Roasted chickpeas include plant-based protein and fiber, which can make you feel full and pleased. They also include iron, which is necessary for the transport of oxygen throughout the body. Furthermore, chickpeas include vitamins and minerals that are necessary for excellent health.

2. Hummus with vegetable sticks

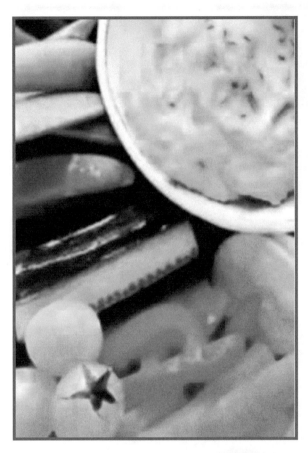

Veggie sticks with hummus are a traditional and filling snack suitable for any occasion. It's simple to make, doesn't require any cooking, and is loaded with nutrients. You may dip a variety of bright veggies, making this a visually appealing and enjoyable alternative for both children and adults.

- ❖ **Preparation time: 5** minutes
- ❖ **Cooking time:** 0 minutes
- ❖ **Total time:** 5 minutes

Ingredients:

- ❖ 1 container (16 oz) of hummus, either store-bought or homemade
- ❖ 3 carrots, peeled and chopped into sticks
- ❖ 3 celery stalks (cut into sticks)
- ❖ Cut one red, yellow, or orange bell pepper into sticks.
- ❖ 1 cucumber, peeled and cut into sticks
- ❖ 1 small head of broccoli with florets chopped into bite-sized pieces (optional)
- ❖ Cherry tomatoes (optional).
- ❖ Snap peas (optional).

Instructions:

- ❖ Wash and prepare the veggies. Cut them into sticks or bite-sized pieces, whatever you want.
- ❖ Place the veggies on a tray or serving dish.
- ❖ Place the hummus jar in the center of the dish, or serve it in separate bowls for dipping.
- ❖ This dish makes roughly four servings.

Nutritional Information: (Per Serving)

- ❖ **Calories:** 170.
- ❖ **Carbohydrate:** 20 grams
- ❖ **Fat:** 8 g
- ❖ **Protein:** 5 grams.
- ❖ **Vitamin A:** 40% of the Daily Value
- ❖ **Vitamin C:** 25 percent DV
- ❖ **Fiber:** 3 grams.

Cooking Tips:

- ❖ To add a fun touch, make a rainbow tray with various colored vegetables.
- ❖ If you're preparing ahead of time, keep the vegetable sticks in an airtight jar in the fridge for up to three days. Hummus may be kept separate for up to a week.
- ❖ Want to add more flavor? Season the veggies with olive oil, balsamic vinegar, or lemon juice.
- ❖ For a more substantial snack, pair the vegetable sticks and hummus with whole-wheat pita bread or crackers.

Health Benefits:

Veggie sticks with hummus are high in vitamins, minerals, and fiber. Here's a summary of some of the main health benefits:

- ❖ Vegetables provide important vitamins, minerals, and antioxidants.
- ❖ Hummus, made from chickpeas, is a rich source of plant-based protein and fiber.
- ❖ Its low calorie and fat content make it an ideal snack for weight management.
- ❖ Fiber promotes digestive health and helps you feel fuller for longer.
- ❖ Portable and handy, ideal for on-the-go munching.

3. Dark Chocolate and Walnut Bites

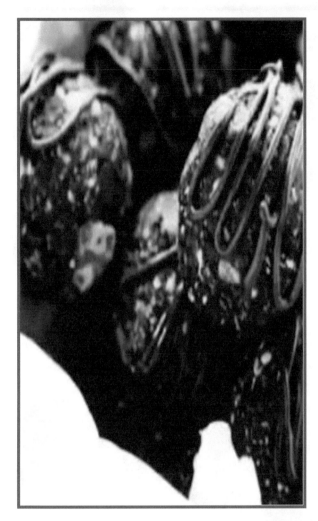

Dark Chocolate and Walnut Bites are a tasty and nutritious snack that will satisfy your sweet desire.

They are high in protein, fiber, and healthy fats from walnuts and dark chocolate, making them an excellent choice for on-the-go energy. They're also very easy to create and don't require any baking!

❖ **Preparation time:** 10 minutes
❖ **Cooking time:** 0 minutes
❖ **Total time:** 10 minutes

Ingredients:

❖ 1 cup rolled oats.
❖ 1/2 cup chopped walnuts.
❖ 1/4 cup unsweetened cocoa powder.
❖ 1/4 cup honey or maple syrup
❖ 1/4 cup nut butter (almond, peanut, or cashew)
❖ Optional: ¼ cup chopped dried fruit (such as raisins, cranberries, or cherries).
❖ Pinch of salt.
❖ 1 cup dark chocolate chips. (melted)

Instructions:

❖ In a large mixing bowl, combine the rolled oats, chopped walnuts, cocoa powder, honey, nut butter, and dried fruit (if desired).
❖ Stir until the ingredients are fully incorporated and a sticky dough forms.
❖ Add the melted dark chocolate chips and gently stir in until just combined.
❖ Line a baking sheet with parchment paper.

- ❖ Scoop out the dough with a spoon or your hands and roll it into bite-size balls. Place them on the prepared baking sheet.
- ❖ Refrigerate for at least 30 minutes, or until the chocolate has set.

Serving Size: This dish makes around 12-15 nibbles.

Nutritional Information (per Serving)

- ❖ **Calories:** 250
- ❖ **Carbohydrate:** 25 grams
- ❖ **Fat:** 12g
- ❖ **Protein:** 5 grams.
- ❖ **Vitamin E:** 4mg (27% of the daily value).
- ❖ **Fiber:** 2 grams

Cooking Tips:

- ❖ Dark chocolate with a greater cacao content (70% or above) will provide a deeper chocolate flavor.
- ❖ If the dough is too sticky, add one additional tablespoon of rolled oats.
- ❖ You may replace the walnuts with other chopped nuts like almonds, pecans, or hazelnuts.
- ❖ Get creative with your add-ins! Try adding chopped dates, shredded coconut, or micro chocolate chips.

Health Benefits:

- ❖ Dark chocolate contains antioxidants and may benefit heart health.
- ❖ Walnuts are high in protein, healthy fats, and fiber, making them a filling and satisfying snack.
- ❖ This dish is a terrific source of energy and may help you stay focused all day.

4. Apple Slices with Peanut Butter

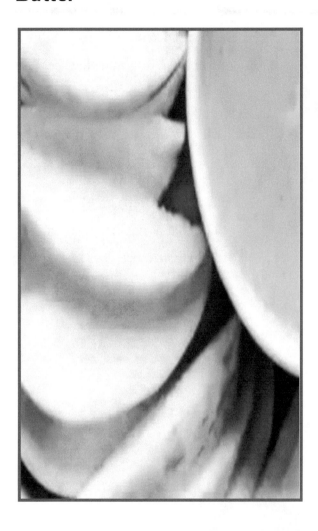

Apple slices with peanut butter are a timeless traditional snack suitable for individuals of all ages. It's high in healthy fats, fiber, and vitamins, making it both nutritional and enjoyable.

- ❖ **Preparation time:** 5 minutes
- ❖ **Cooking time:** 0 minutes
- ❖ **Total time:** 5 minutes

Ingredients:

- ❖ 1 apple (whatever kind you like, although tart apples like Granny Smith combine nicely with peanut butter)
- ❖ 2 tablespoons peanut butter (creamy or chunky, whatever you want)
- ❖ Lemon juice (optional, to avoid browning)

Instructions:

- ❖ Wash the apples and cut them into wedges. You may core the apple first, or leave it in for a thicker slice.
- ❖ To avoid browning, mix the apple slices in a basin with a tablespoon of lemon juice.
- ❖ Spread peanut butter on the apple slices or serve them as dip.

Serving size: This recipe yields one serving.

Nutritional Information: (Based on a granny smith apple and two tablespoons of creamy peanut butter)

- ❖ **Calories:** 190
- ❖ **Carbohydrates:** 25g
- ❖ **Fat:** 8g

- ❖ **Protein:** 4 grams
- ❖ **Vitamin C:** 8%. DV
- ❖ **Fiber:** 4 grams

Cooking Tips:

- ❖ For a fun twist, experiment with other nut butters such as almond butter or cashew butter.
- ❖ If you don't have fresh apples, pre-sliced apples will do just fine.
- ❖ Want to add some more crunch? Sprinkle granola or chopped nuts over the peanut butter.
- ❖ To keep the apple slices from browning ahead of time, place them in a jar lined with a moist paper towel.

Health Benefits:

- ❖ Apples include fiber, which aids digestion and keeps you feeling full.
- ❖ Peanut butter is a nutritious fat that contains protein and other minerals.
- ❖ This snack contains vitamin C, which is essential for immunological function.
- ❖ Apple slices with peanut butter are a nutritious and delicious snack that will help you meet your daily fruit, healthy fat, and fiber requirements.

5. Blueberry Almond Bars

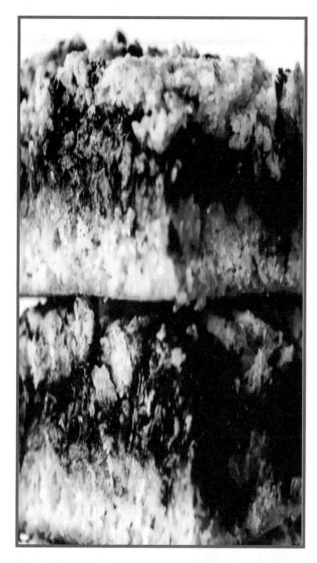

These delicious snacks are packed with fresh blueberries and nutty almond flavor. They make an excellent quick and tasty snack or dessert and can be prepared in about an hour.

- ❖ **Preparation time:** 10 minutes
- ❖ **Cooking Time:** 30–35 minutes
- ❖ **Total Time:** 40-45 minutes

Ingredients:

- ❖ 1 1/2 cups all-purpose flour
- ❖ ¾ cup rolled oats (old-fashioned is best)
- ❖ 1/2 cup granulated sugar.
- ❖ ½ cup unsalted butter, softened
- ❖ ½ teaspoon almond essence
- ❖ ½ teaspoon salt.
- ❖ 2 cups of fresh blueberries.
- ❖ 1/2 cup sliced almonds.

Instructions:

- ❖ Preheat the oven to 350°F (175°C). Line an 8x8-inch baking pan with parchment paper for easy removal.
- ❖ In a large bowl, mix the flour, oats, sugar, and salt. Using a pastry cutter or two forks, work in the softened butter until it resembles coarse crumbs. Stir in the almond extract.
- ❖ Set aside about 1 cup of the crumb mixture for the topping. Spread the leftover dough equally in the bottom of the prepared pan.
- ❖ Spread the fresh blueberries equally throughout the flattened dough.
- ❖ Sprinkle the blueberries with the leftover crumb mixture and sliced

almonds. Gently press down to adhere somewhat.

- ❖ Bake for 30-35 minutes, or until the sides turn golden brown and the filling bubbles.
- ❖ Allow to cool fully in the pan on a wire rack before cutting into bars.

Serving size: 12 bars.

Nutrition Facts: (per bar)

- ❖ **Calories:** 250
- ❖ **Carbohydrates:** 35g
- ❖ **Fat:** 10g
- ❖ **Protein:** 4g
- ❖ **Vitamin C:** 10% DV (from blueberries)
- ❖ **Fiber:** 2 grams

Cooking Tips:

- ❖ To enhance the flavor, toast the sliced almonds in a dry pan over medium heat for a few minutes until fragrant before adding to the topping.
- ❖ If your blueberries are really juicy, mix them with a spoonful of cornstarch before adding them to the bars. This will help keep the filling from being too sloppy.
- ❖ Do not overbake the bars. They are done when the edges are golden brown and the filling bubbles but does not overflow.

Health Benefits:

- ❖ Blueberries are high in antioxidants and vitamin C, which can help your immune system function better.
- ❖ Almonds are an excellent source of protein, fiber, and healthy fat.
- ❖ Oatmeal is a complete grain that delivers continuous energy and may help decrease cholesterol levels.

6. Almond and Walnut Mixture

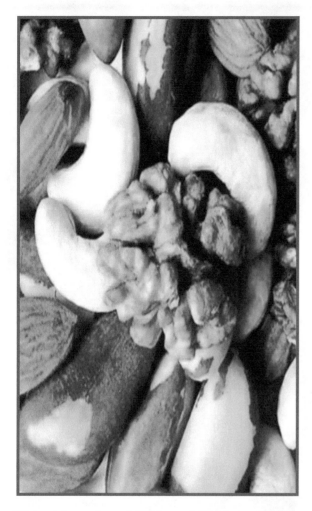

This Almond and Walnut Mix is a simple yet delicious snack mix that blends the pleasing crunch of almonds with the rich, nutty taste of walnuts. This handcrafted mix is ideal for on-the-go energy or as a nutritious addition to salads and yogurt parfaits. It has no added sweets or preservatives, making it a guilt-free pleasure.

❖ **Preparation time:** 5 minutes
❖ **Cooking time:** 0 minutes
❖ **Total time:** 5 minutes

Ingredients:

❖ 1 cup raw almonds.
❖ 1 cup raw walnuts.
❖ 1/2 teaspoon sea salt (optional)

Instructions:

❖ In a large basin, add the almonds and walnuts.
❖ If desired, season with sea salt and toss to coat.
❖ Keep in an airtight jar at room temperature for up to a week.

Serving Size: 1/2 cup.

Nutritional Information (per Serving)

❖ **Calories:** 164
❖ **Carbs:** 6g
❖ **Fat:** 14g
❖ **Protein:** 6 grams.
❖ **Vitamin E:** 7mg (47% DV).
❖ **Fiber:** 1.5 grams.

Cooking Tips:

❖ For a more complex flavor, roast the almonds and walnuts for 5-7 minutes at 350°F (175°C). Let cool fully before storing.

❖ For a sweeter flavor, consider adding dried fruit such as cranberries or chopped dates.

❖ Experiment with various nut pairings! Pecans, cashews, and pistachios would all make excellent additions.

Health Benefits:

❖ Almonds and walnuts are both high in healthy fats, protein, and fiber, making them filling and satisfying.

❖ They are also high in vitamin E, an antioxidant essential for cell health.

❖ Nuts in your diet may help lower your risk of heart disease, type 2 diabetes, and several malignancies.

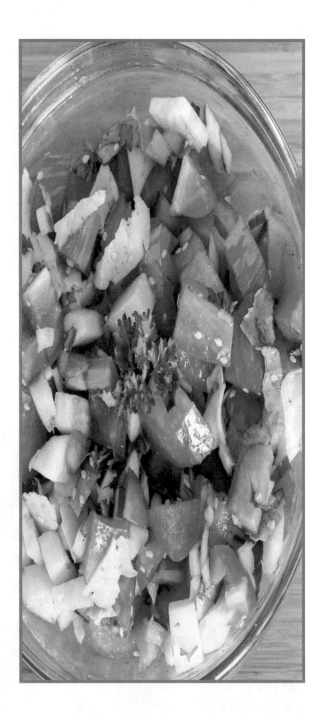

7. Spinach & Artichoke Dip

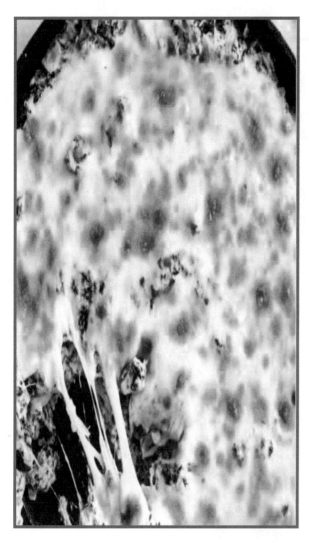

This creamy and delicious Spinach and Artichoke Dip is a fan favorite! It's easy to create and completely adaptable, making it ideal for parties, snacks, or a relaxed night in.

- ❖ **Preparation time:** 10 minutes
- ❖ **Cook time:** 20-25 minutes.
- ❖ **Total time:** 30–35 minutes

Ingredients:

- ❖ 8 oz cream cheese, softened
- ❖ ¼ cup mayonnaise
- ❖ 1/4 cup sour cream.
- ❖ Mince 1 garlic clove and use 1/2 teaspoon dried basil.
- ❖ ¼ teaspoon dried oregano.
- ❖ Add salt and pepper to taste.
- ❖ 1 (14 ounce) can of artichoke hearts, drained and diced
- ❖ 1/2 cup frozen chopped spinach, thawed and drained
- ❖ 1/2 cup shredded mozzarella cheese.
- ❖ ¼ cup grated Parmesan

Instructions:

- ❖ Preheat the oven to 350°F (175°C). Lightly butter a small baking dish (4-5 cups).
- ❖ In a medium bowl, whisk together softened cream cheese, mayonnaise, sour cream, garlic, basil, oregano, salt, and pepper until smooth and creamy.
- ❖ Gently fold in the chopped artichoke hearts, spinach, and mozzarella cheese.

- Pour the mixture into the prepared baking dish. Sprinkle the top with Parmesan cheese.
- Bake for 20-25 minutes, or until bubbling and light golden brown.

Serving Size: This dish makes roughly six servings.

Nutrition Information: Per serving (based on six portions)

- **Calories:** 300.
- **Carbohydrates:** 10g
- **Fat:** 25g
- **Protein:** 10g.
- **Vitamin A:** 40%. DV
- **Calcium:** 20%. DV
- **Fiber:** 2 grams.

Cooking Tips:

- Full-fat sour cream and cream cheese provide a fuller taste.
- To make the dip hotter, add a sprinkle of red pepper flakes or diced fresh jalapenos.
- If the dip appears overly thick, add a tablespoon of milk or broth to dilute it.
- Leftover dip may be refrigerated in an airtight container for up to three days. Reheat gently in the microwave or oven until heated through.

Health Benefits:

- Spinach contains vitamins A, K, iron, and folate.
- Artichokes are a wonderful source of fiber and antioxidants.
- Cream and mozzarella cheese include calcium and protein.
- Enjoy this tasty and adaptable Spinach and Artichoke Dip!

Chapter 5

Fresh and Vibrant Salads and Soup

1. Butternut Squash and Carrot Soup

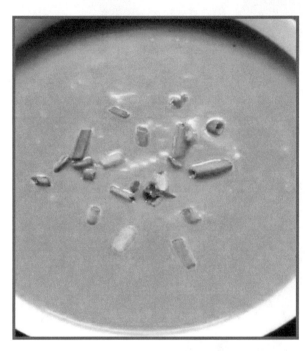

This creamy and savory soup is an excellent way to experience the flavors of autumn. Butternut squash and carrots are roasted to bring out their natural sweetness, then combined with broth and spices for a hearty and fulfilling supper.

- ❖ **Preparation time:** 15 minutes
- ❖ **Cooking time:** 40 minutes
- ❖ **Total time:** 55 minutes

Ingredients:

- ❖ 1 medium butternut squash (about 2 pounds), peeled, seeded, and diced.
- ❖ Four carrots, peeled and sliced
- ❖ 1 tablespoon of olive oil.
- ❖ Chop one medium onion and mince three cloves of garlic.
- ❖ 4 cups veggie broth.
- ❖ 1 teaspoon ground cumin.
- ❖ 1/2 teaspoon of ground ginger.
- ❖ Add salt and freshly ground black pepper to taste.
- ❖ 1/2 cup heavy cream (optional; for a richer soup)
- ❖ Chopped fresh parsley for garnish (optional).

Instructions:

- ❖ Preheat the oven to 400° F (200° C). Line a baking sheet with parchment paper.
- ❖ Toss the butternut squash and carrots with olive oil and lay them out on the

baking sheet. Roast for 30 to 35 minutes, or until soft and gently browned.

❖ While the veggies roast, preheat a large saucepan over medium heat. Cook for 5 minutes, or until the onion has softened. Stir in the garlic and simmer for another minute.

❖ Place the roasted veggies, vegetable broth, cumin, and ginger in the pot. Bring to a boil, then decrease the heat and simmer for 15 minutes.

❖ Using an immersion blender or transferring the soup to a blender, mix until smooth. Season with salt and pepper to taste.

❖ If using, stir in the heavy cream and heat until thoroughly combined.

❖ Serve hot and sprinkle with chopped fresh parsley (optional).

Serving size: 4-6 servings

Nutritional Information (per Serving)

❖ **Calories:** 200-250 (depends on whether heavy cream is used)

❖ **Carbohydrates:** 30-35g

❖ **Fat:** 5-10 g

❖ **Protein:** 4-5 g

❖ **Vitamin A** is very high (thanks to the butternut squash and carrots).

❖ **Fiber:** 5–7 grams.

Cooking Tips:

❖ Roast the veggies with a sprig of fresh thyme to add a deeper taste.

❖ To make the soup vegan, skip the heavy cream and substitute coconut milk.

❖ Refrigerate leftovers in an airtight jar for up to three days.

Health Benefits:

❖ Butternut squash and carrots are high in vitamins and minerals, such as vitamin A, C, and potassium.

❖ This soup has plenty of fiber, which aids digestion and keeps you full.

❖ The soup's smoothness may be gratifying, making it a suitable option for those looking to lose weight.

2. Tomato Basil Soup with Whole-Grain Croutons

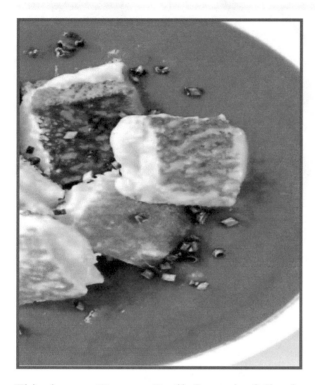

This hearty Tomato Basil Soup is full of fresh flavor and works nicely with homemade whole-grain croutons. It's a simple dish ideal for a fast weeknight supper.

- ❖ **Preparation time:** 10 minutes
- ❖ **Cook time:** 30 minutes
- ❖ **Total time:** 40 minutes

Ingredients:

For the soup:

- ❖ 1 tablespoon of olive oil.

- ❖ 1 red onion, chopped
- ❖ 2 garlic cloves, minced
- ❖ 2 (28-ounce) cans of crushed tomatoes.
- ❖ For 4 cups vegetable broth, add 1/2 cup chopped fresh basil or 1 tablespoon dried basil.
- ❖ 1 teaspoon of dried oregano.
- ❖ 1/2 teaspoon of red pepper flakes (optional)
- ❖ Add salt and freshly ground black pepper to taste.

For whole-grain croutons:

- ❖ 2 cups of whole wheat bread, sliced into 1 inch cubes.
- ❖ 2 tablespoons of olive oil.
- ❖ 1/2 teaspoon dried thyme.
- ❖ 1/4 teaspoon of garlic powder.
- ❖ Add salt and freshly ground black pepper to taste.

Instructions:

- ❖ Make the croutons: Preheat the oven to 375° Fahrenheit (190° Celsius). In a large mixing bowl, combine bread cubes, olive oil, thyme, garlic powder, salt, and pepper. Place the cubes on a baking sheet in a single layer and bake for 15-20 minutes, or until golden brown and toasted. Set aside.

❖ Make the soup: In a large saucepan, heat the olive oil over medium heat. Cook until the onion softens, which should take around 5 minutes. Stir in the garlic and simmer for another minute.

❖ Combine the crushed tomatoes, vegetable broth, basil, oregano, and red pepper flakes (if using). Bring to a boil, then decrease the heat and simmer for 20 minutes.

❖ Using an immersion blender, purée the soup in the pot until smooth, or transfer to a blender and puree in stages. Season with salt and pepper to taste.

❖ Ladle the soup into bowls and top with croutons. Enjoy!

Serving Size: Four servings

Nutritional Information: Per serving (excluding croutons):

❖ **Calories:** 200
❖ **Carbohydrate:** 25 grams
❖ **Fat:** 5 g
❖ **Protein:** 5 grams

❖ **Vitamin A:** 20% of the Daily Value
❖ **Vitamin C:** 30%. DV
❖ **Fiber:** 3 grams

Cooking Tips:

❖ To make the soup richer, add a dash of heavy cream or coconut milk before serving.

❖ If you don't have fresh basil, use 1 tablespoon dried basil.

❖ To make the soup vegan, use vegetable broth and leave out the cheese.

❖ Croutons can be prepared ahead of time and kept in an airtight container for up to a week.

Health Benefits:

❖ Tomatoes are rich in vitamins A, C, and potassium.

❖ Basil is rich in antioxidants.

❖ Whole wheat bread is high in fiber.

❖ This soup is a nutritious and comforting dinner ideal for a cold day.

3. Lentil And Vegetable Soup

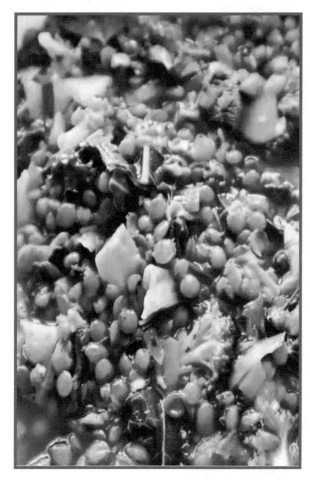

Lentil and vegetable soup is a tasty and healthy dish suitable for any occasion. The lentils provide protein and fiber, while the veggies supply vitamins and minerals. Plus, it's robust and nourishing, making it ideal for a cold winter day or a light lunch.

- ❖ **Preparation time:** 10 minutes
- ❖ **Cook time:** 30 minutes
- ❖ **Total time:** 40 minutes

Ingredients:

- ❖ 1 tablespoon of olive oil.
- ❖ 1 onion, chopped
- ❖ To prepare, cut two carrots, two celery stalks, and mince two garlic cloves.
- ❖ 1 teaspoon ground cumin.
- ❖ 1 teaspoon dried thyme.
- ❖ 1 (28-ounce) can of diced tomatoes, undrained.
- ❖ 1 cup brown lentils, washed
- ❖ 4 cups veggie broth.
- ❖ 1 cup water.
- ❖ 1 teaspoon salt.
- ❖ A pinch of red pepper flakes (optional)
- ❖ 1 cup of chopped kale or spinach.
- ❖ 1 tablespoon of lemon juice (optional)

Instructions:

- ❖ In a large saucepan, heat the olive oil over medium heat. Cook the onion, carrots, and celery for approximately 5 minutes, or until softened.
- ❖ Add the garlic, cumin, and thyme and simmer for another minute, or until fragrant.

- Add the chopped tomatoes, lentils, vegetable broth, water, salt, and red pepper flakes (if using). Bring to a boil, then lower the heat and simmer for 25-30 minutes, or until the lentils are cooked but still maintain their form.
- Add the kale or spinach and simmer for about 1 minute, or until wilted.
- Remove from heat and add lemon juice (if using).

Serving Size: Four servings

Nutrition Facts: (per serving)

- **Calories:** 300
- **Carbohydrate:** 40 grams
- **Fat:** 8g
- **Protein:** 15 grams
- **Vitamin A:** 25% of the Daily Value
- **Vitamin C:** 30%. DV
- **Fiber:** 8 grams

Cooking Tips:

- To make the soup thicker, mash some of the cooked lentils against the pot's side with a fork.
- If you don't have fresh kale or spinach, you may use 1 cup frozen peas. Add them in the final few minutes of cooking.
- You may add other veggies to this soup, such as zucchini, potatoes, or green beans.

Health Benefits:

- Lentils contain plant-based protein and fiber, which can make you feel full and pleased.
- Vegetables include vitamins, minerals, and antioxidants that are necessary for optimum health.
- This soup is also high in vitamin A, which is essential for clear vision and healthy skin.
- The fiber in this soup can assist to regulate digestion and improve intestinal health.
- This lentil and vegetable soup is a tasty and nutritious dinner that is simple to prepare. It's an excellent supplement to any healthy diet due to its high protein, fiber, vitamin, and mineral content.

4. Mixed greens, berries, and nuts

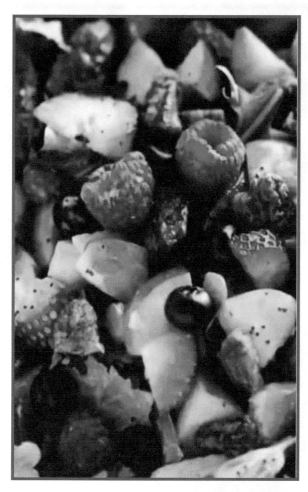

This Mixed Greens with Berries and Nuts salad is overflowing with fresh tastes and textures and makes an excellent light lunch or side dish. The richness of the berries balances the earthy greens, and the crunch of the almonds provides a delightful contrast.

- ❖ **Preparation time:** 5 minutes
- ❖ **Cooking time:** 0 minutes
- ❖ **Total time:** 5 minutes

Ingredients:

- ❖ 5 ounces mixed greens (spring mix, romaine, spinach, etc.)
- ❖ 1 cup fresh, sliced strawberries
- ❖ 1/2 cup of fresh blueberries.
- ❖ 1/2 cup of fresh raspberries.
- ❖ 1/4 cup crumbled feta cheese (optional).
- ❖ 1/4 cup chopped walnuts, pecans, or almonds.

For dressing:

- ❖ 2 tablespoons of olive oil.
- ❖ 1 tablespoon of lemon juice.
- ❖ 1/2 teaspoon honey.
- ❖ Add salt and pepper to taste.

Instructions:

- ❖ Wash and dry your mixed greens. Place them in a big basin.
- ❖ Hull and slice the strawberries. Add them to the bowl beside the blueberries and raspberries.
- ❖ If used, scatter the feta over the salad.
- ❖ Toast the nuts in a dry pan over medium heat for 5 minutes, or until aromatic. Pay special attention to

avoid burning. Alternatively, omit the toasting for a milder flavor. Roughly cut the nuts and scatter them over the salad.

❖ In a small jar or dish, combine olive oil, lemon juice, honey, salt, and pepper.

❖ Drizzle the dressing over the salad right before serving. Toss lightly to coat.

Serving size per recipe: 2 servings.

Nutrition Facts: (Per Serving)

❖ **Calories:** 300
❖ **Carbohydrates:** 25g
❖ **Fat:** 15g
❖ **Protein:** 5 grams
❖ **Vitamin C:** 60% of the Daily Value (DV).
❖ **Fiber:** 4 grams

Cooking Tips:

❖ For a sweeter salad, substitute dried fruits such as cranberries or chopped dates for, or in addition to, fresh berries.

❖ Toasted nuts have a richer flavor, but you may avoid toasting if you prefer a milder taste.

❖ Leftover salad can be refrigerated for up to one day. However, the dressing can wilt the greens, so keep it separate and add it before serving.

Health Benefits:

❖ Mixed greens contain vitamins, minerals, and antioxidants.

❖ Berries include antioxidants and Vitamin C, which can help your immune system.

❖ Nuts provide healthy fats, protein, and fiber, which help you feel full and content.

❖ This salad is low-calorie and low-carb, making it ideal for people managing their weight.

5. Kale and Quinoa Salad with Lemon Dressing

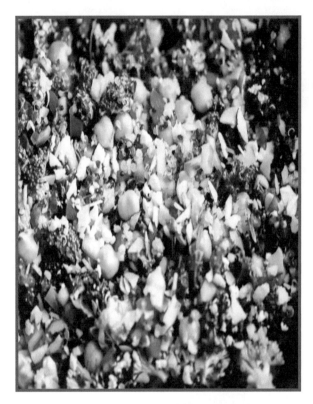

This colorful Kale and Quinoa Salad with Lemon Dressing is loaded with protein, minerals, and fiber. It's a light and refreshing salad, ideal for a nutritious lunch or side dish. The delicious lemon dressing balances the earthy kale and nutty quinoa nicely. Additionally, it is entirely configurable! Feel free to include your favorite chopped veggies, fruits, nuts, or seeds.

- ❖ **Preparation time:** 10 minutes
- ❖ **Cooking time:** 15 minutes for quinoa
- ❖ **Total time:** 25 minutes

Ingredients:

- ❖ 1 cup dried quinoa, washed
- ❖ 1 3/4 cups water/vegetable broth
- ❖ 5 cups chopped kale (ribs removed).
- ❖ 1/2 cup halved cherry tomatoes
- ❖ 1 thinly sliced cucumber
- ❖ 1 sliced red bell pepper, and 1 (15-ounce) can drained and washed chickpeas.
- ❖ 1/2 cup crumbled feta cheese (optional).
- ❖ Toasted 1/4 cup sliced almonds with lemon dressing.
- ❖ 6 tablespoons of extra-virgin olive oil
- ❖ 3 tablespoons of lemon juice.
- ❖ 2 tablespoons chopped shallots or red onions
- ❖ 1 teaspoon of honey or maple syrup.
- ❖ 1/2 teaspoon dijon mustard (optional)
- ❖ Add salt and freshly ground black pepper to taste.

Instructions:

- ❖ Cook the quinoa: In a saucepan, mix the washed quinoa with water or broth. Bring to a boil, then decrease heat, cover, and simmer for 15 minutes, or until the quinoa is fluffy and fully cooked. Remove from heat and let it fluff for 5 minutes.

- ❖ Preparing the salad: While the quinoa is cooking, gently massage the kale in a large bowl with olive oil to soften it. Combine the cherry tomatoes, cucumber, red pepper, chickpeas, and feta cheese (if using).
- ❖ Prepare the lemon dressing: In a small mixing bowl, combine the olive oil, lemon juice, shallots, honey, Dijon mustard (if using), salt, and pepper.
- ❖ Assemble the salad: Once the quinoa is cooked, place it in a salad dish with the remaining ingredients. Pour the lemon dressing over the salad and toss to coat evenly.
- ❖ Garnish the salad with toasted almonds and serve immediately.

Serving size: Each dish yields four servings.

Nutrition Facts: (per serving)

- ❖ **Calories:** 400
- ❖ **Carbohydrates:** 50g
- ❖ **Fat:** 15g.
- ❖ **Protein:** 10 grams.
- ❖ **Vitamin A:** 20% of the Daily Value

- ❖ **Vitamin C:** 40%. DV
- ❖ **Fiber:** 5 grams

Cooking Tips:

- ❖ To toast the almonds, place them on a baking sheet and bake in a 350°F oven for 5-7 minutes, or until golden brown. To avoid burns, keep a tight eye on them.
- ❖ If you don't have fresh shallots, you may use red onion.
- ❖ For a vegan salad, leave off the feta cheese.
- ❖ This salad is considerably more tasty after chilling for at least 30 minutes before serving. The tastes will have time to come together.

Health Benefits:

- ❖ Kale is a superfood full of vitamins, minerals, and antioxidants.
- ❖ Quinoa is a complete protein, which means it includes all nine important amino acids your body needs.
- ❖ This salad has plenty of fiber, which keeps you full and content.
- ❖ The lemon dressing adds flavor to your salad while remaining light and nutritious.

6. Spinach and Strawberry Salad

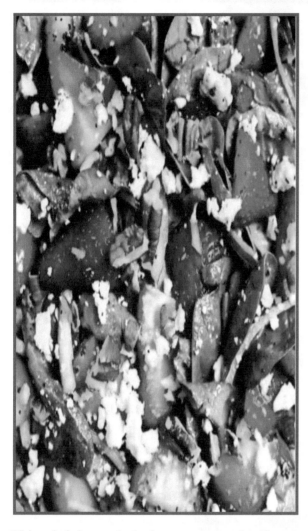

This bright salad has sweet, luscious strawberries and crisp spinach leaves. It's the ideal refreshing side dish or light meal, filled with flavor and minerals.

- ❖ **Preparation time:** 5 minutes
- ❖ **Cooking time:** 0 minutes
- ❖ **Total time:** 5 minutes

Ingredients:

- ❖ 2 bunches of fresh spinach, cleaned and cut into bite-sized pieces (about. 5 oz)
- ❖ 1 pound of fresh strawberries, hulled and sliced.
- ❖ 1/2 cup crumbled feta cheese (optional).
- ❖ 1/4 cup chopped walnuts or pecans (optional).

For the poppy seed dressing:

- ❖ 1/4 cup olive oil.
- ❖ 2 teaspoons of white balsamic vinegar (or normal balsamic vinegar).
- ❖ 1 tablespoon honey
- ❖ 1 teaspoon Dijon mustard.
- ❖ 1/2 teaspoon of poppy seeds.
- ❖ Add salt and freshly ground black pepper to taste.

Instructions:

- ❖ In a large bowl, mix the spinach and strawberries.
- ❖ In a separate mixing bowl, combine the olive oil, balsamic vinegar,

honey, Dijon mustard, poppy seeds, salt, and pepper.

- ❖ Pour the dressing over the salad and toss to coat.
- ❖ Add the feta cheese and walnuts or pecans (if using) and mix again.
- ❖ Serve immediately.

Serving Size: Two servings

Nutritional Information (per Serving)

- ❖ **Calories:** 250
- ❖ **Carbohydrates:** 20g
- ❖ **Fat:** 12g.
- ❖ **Protein:** 5 grams.
- ❖ **Vitamin C:** 140%. DV
- ❖ **Fiber:** 4 grams.

Cooking Tips:

- ❖ Instead of only spinach, try a variety of lettuces to make your salad more tasty. Arugula, romaine, and butter lettuce would all work nicely.
- ❖ If you don't have fresh strawberries, you may substitute frozen strawberries that have been thawed and dried.
- ❖ To keep the strawberries from browning too rapidly, mix them with a little amount of lemon juice before adding them to the salad.

Health Benefits:

- ❖ Spinach is rich in vitamins A, C, and K, as well as iron and folate.
- ❖ Strawberries are rich in vitamin C, fiber, and manganese.
- ❖ This salad is a nutritious and pleasant way to receive your daily serving of fruits and veggies.

7. Mushroom & Barley Stew

Ingredients:

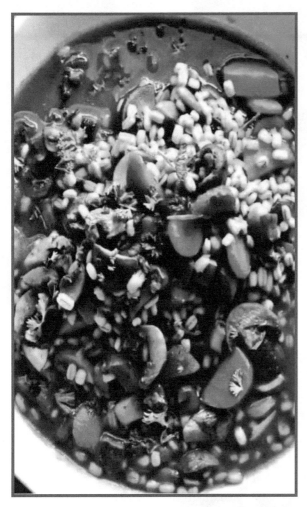

- ❖ 2 tablespoons of olive oil.
- ❖ 1 yellow onion, chopped
- ❖ To prepare, dice 2 carrots, 2 celery stalks, and mince 4 garlic cloves.
- ❖ 1 pound of sliced mushrooms (cremini, portobello, white button, or a mixture)
- ❖ 1/2 cup pearl barley.
- ❖ 6 cups vegetable broth, 1 tablespoon soy sauce (or tamari for gluten-free options).
- ❖ 1 teaspoon dried thyme.
- ❖ 1/2 teaspoon dried rosemary.
- ❖ 1 bay leaf.
- ❖ Add salt and freshly ground black pepper to taste.
- ❖ Freshly cut parsley for garnish (optional)

This rich mushroom and barley stew is a soothing and filling dinner ideal for a nice night in. It contains savory mushrooms, delicate barley, and a thick vegetable broth, making it a tasty and nutritious vegetarian alternative.

- ❖ **Preparation time:** 10 minutes
- ❖ **Cooking time:** 40 to 50 minutes
- ❖ **Total time:** 50-60 minutes

Instructions:

- ❖ In a big saucepan or Dutch oven, bring the olive oil to a medium heat. Combine the onions, carrots, and celery. Cook for 5–7 minutes, or until softened.
- ❖ Stir in the garlic and simmer for another minute, until fragrant.

- Cook the sliced mushrooms for 5-7 minutes, or until tender and golden.
- Combine the pearl barley, vegetable broth, soy sauce, thyme, rosemary, and bay leaf. Bring to a boil, then lower to a low heat, cover, and cook for 40-50 minutes, until the barley is soft and chewy.
- Season with salt and pepper to taste. Remove the bay leaf before serving.
- Garnish with fresh chopped parsley if preferred.

Serving size: 4-6 servings

Nutrition Facts: (per serving)

- **Calories:** 300–350
- **Carbohydrates:** 40 to 45 grams
- **Fat:** 10-12 g
- **Protein:** 15-20 g
- **Vitamin C:** 10% Daily Value (DV)
- **Fiber:** 5–7 grams

Cooking Tips:

- Instead of adding all of the mushrooms at once, brown them in batches for a deeper taste. This will assist them release their juices, resulting in a more caramelized taste.
- If you don't have mixed mushrooms, you may substitute any variety of mushroom you choose, such as white button, cremini, or portobello.
- You may modify the amount of vegetable broth in your stew based on how thick you want it.
- To make this stew vegan, simply leave out the soy sauce and use vegetable stock instead of chicken broth.
- Refrigerate leftovers in an airtight jar for up to three days.

Health Benefits:

- Mushrooms are rich in vitamins, minerals, and antioxidants.
- Barley is a complete grain rich in fiber, which aids digestion and keeps you full.
- This stew is high in plant-based protein, making it suitable for both vegetarians and vegans.

Chapter 6

Main Dishes Recipes

Fish and Seafood

1. Tuna & White Bean Salad

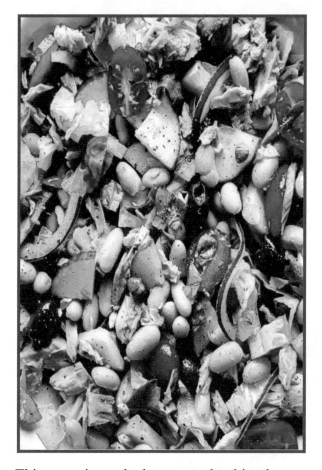

This protein-packed tuna and white bean salad makes a delightful and filling lunch. It's also really adaptable; you can have it on sandwiches, wraps, or lettuce cups, or as a side dish. Plus, it takes only 15 minutes to put together!

❖ **Preparation time:** 5 minutes
❖ **Cooking time:** 0 minutes
❖ **Total time:** 15 minutes

Ingredients:

❖ 1 (15-ounce) can of cannellini beans, washed and drained
❖ 1 (5-ounce) canned tuna packed in water, drained
❖ 1/2 cup diced red onion
❖ 1/4 cup chopped fresh parsley.
❖ 2 tablespoons of olive oil.
❖ 1 tablespoon of lemon juice.
❖ 1/2 teaspoon of dried oregano.
❖ 1/4 teaspoon salt and 1/4 teaspoon freshly ground black pepper.

Instructions:

❖ In a medium bowl, mix together the cannellini beans, tuna, red onion, and parsley.

- In a separate dish, mix the olive oil, lemon juice, oregano, salt, and pepper.
- Toss the salad ingredients with the dressing until well coated.
- Serve immediately or refrigerate for at least 30 minutes to let the flavors combine.

Serving size per recipe: 2 servings.

Nutritional Information:

- **Calories:** 300.
- *Carbohydrates:* 30g
- **Fat:** 10g.
- **Protein:** 20 grams
- **Vitamin C:** 6%. DV
- **Fiber:** 5 grams.

Cooking Tips:

- To make the salad creamier, mash some of the cannellini beans before adding them to the dish.
- If you don't have fresh parsley, use 1 teaspoon dried parsley.
- Add more chopped veggies to the salad, such as celery, cucumber, or bell peppers.
- If you desire a stronger tuna flavor, use tuna packed in oil rather than water. Just make sure you drain the oil before adding the tuna to the salad.

Health Benefits:

- Tuna and white bean salad is high in lean protein and fiber, which can make you feel full and content. It also contains beneficial fats from olive oil, which can benefit heart health. In addition, the salad contains vitamin C and fiber, which are beneficial to general health.

2. Grilled Shrimp and Quinoa Salad

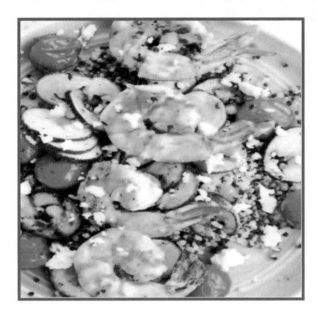

This recipe is a delicious and nutritious blend of protein-rich grilled prawns with a fluffy quinoa salad. It's ideal for a light lunch, a hearty dinner, or a cool summer feast.

- ❖ **Preparation time:** 15 minutes
- ❖ **Cook time:** 20 minutes.
- ❖ **Total time:** 35 minutes.

Ingredients:

For the shrimp:

- ❖ 1 pound big peeled and deveined shrimp
- ❖ 2 tablespoons of olive oil.
- ❖ 1 tablespoon of fresh lime juice.
- ❖ 1 teaspoon of chili powder.
- ❖ 1/2 teaspoon of ground cumin
- ❖ 1/4 teaspoon of smoked paprika.
- ❖ 1/4 teaspoon of garlic powder.
- ❖ Add salt and black pepper to taste.

For the quinoa salad:

- ❖ 1 cup uncooked quinoa
- ❖ 1 1/2 cups vegetable broth
- ❖ 1/2 cup diced red bell pepper.
- ❖ 1/2 cup chopped cucumber.
- ❖ 1/4 cup diced red onion
- ❖ 1/4 cup chopped fresh cilantro.
- ❖ 2 tablespoons of olive oil.
- ❖ 1 tablespoon of fresh lime juice.
- ❖ 1/2 teaspoon of ground cumin
- ❖ Add salt and black pepper to taste.

Instructions:

- ❖ Marinate the Shrimp: In a medium bowl, combine the olive oil, lime juice, chili powder, cumin, paprika, garlic powder, salt, and pepper. Add the shrimp and toss to coat. Marinate for at least fifteen minutes.
- ❖ Cook the Quinoa: In a saucepan, mix the quinoa and vegetable stock. Bring to a boil, then decrease heat,

cover, and simmer for 15 minutes, or until the quinoa is fully cooked and fluffy. Remove from heat and let it fluff with a fork for 5 minutes.

❖ Prepare the Salad: In a large mixing bowl, add cooked quinoa, red bell pepper, cucumber, red onion, and cilantro.

❖ Make the Dressing: In a small bowl, combine the olive oil, lime juice, cumin, salt, and pepper.

❖ Grill the Shrimp: Heat a grill or grill pan to medium-high. Grill the shrimp for 2-3 minutes on each side, or until cooked through and opaque.

❖ To assemble the dish, combine the quinoa salad with the dressing. Divide the salad amongst plates and top with grilled shrimp.

Serving size: This recipe makes 4 servings.

Nutritional Information (per Serving)

❖ **Calories:** 400.
❖ **Carbohydrates:** 40g
❖ **Fat:** 15g.
❖ **Protein:** 30 grams.
❖ **Vitamin C:** 10 percent DV
❖ **Fiber:** 4 grams.

Cooking Tips:

❖ To keep the shrimp from sticking to the grill, warm it thoroughly and gently oil the grates before adding them.

❖ If you don't have a grill, saute the shrimp in a heated pan over medium-high heat for a few minutes on each side.

❖ To make the salad hotter, add a sprinkle of cayenne pepper to the dressing.

❖ You may add other veggies to the salad, including chopped corn, black beans, or avocado.

Health Benefits:

❖ Shrimp is a fantastic source of lean protein that is low in calories and fat.

❖ Quinoa is a complete protein, which means it has all nine necessary amino acids. It also contains plenty of fiber and complex carbs.

❖ This meal has plenty of vitamin C, which helps to improve the immune system.

❖ Olive oil contains beneficial lipids that can assist enhance heart health.

3. Baked salmon with garlic and herbs

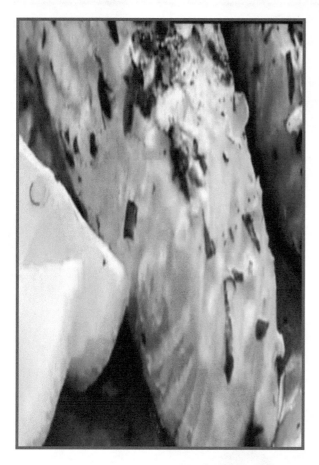

Baked salmon with garlic & herbs is a traditional recipe that is simple to prepare and always impresses. The fish is perfectly cooked, and the garlic and herb butter adds a wonderful taste. This recipe is ideal for a quick and easy weekday supper or a more formal dinner occasion.

- ❖ **Preparation time:** 10 minutes
- ❖ **Cook time:** 15-20 minutes
- ❖ **Total Time:** 25-30 minutes

Ingredients:

- ❖ 2 salmon filets (approx. 6 ounces each).
- ❖ 2 tablespoons unsalted butter, softened.
- ❖ 2 garlic cloves, minced
- ❖ To prepare, chop
- ❖ 1 tablespoon fresh parsley
- ❖ 1 tablespoon fresh dill
- ❖ 1/2 teaspoon dried thyme.
- ❖ 1/2 teaspoon of salt.
- ❖ 1/4 teaspoon of black pepper.
- ❖ 1 lemon sliced (optional)

Instructions:

- ❖ Preheat the oven to 400° F (200° C). Line a baking sheet with parchment paper.
- ❖ Pat the salmon filets dry with paper towels.
- ❖ In a small bowl, mix together the melted butter, garlic, parsley, dill, thyme, salt, and pepper.
- ❖ Place the salmon filets on the prepared baking sheet. Spread the garlic herb butter evenly on top of the fish.
- ❖ Top with lemon slices if desired.

- Bake for 15-20 minutes, or until the salmon is well cooked and readily flaked with a fork.

Serving Size: One salmon filet.

Nutritional Information:

- **Calories:** 400.
- **Carbohydrate:** 0g
- **Fat:** 30g
- **Protein:** 40 grams.
- **Vitamin D:** 500 IU (125% DV).
- **Omega-3 fatty acids:** 2,000 mg.
- **Fiber:** 0 grams.

Cooking Tips:

- For additional crispy skin, broil the salmon for the last minute or two of cooking time.
- If you don't have fresh herbs, use 1 teaspoon dried herbs instead.
- To see if the salmon is cooked through, stick a fork into the thickest section of the filet. The salmon should flake easily and remain opaque throughout.

Health Benefits:

- Salmon is an excellent source of lean protein, healthy fats, and essential vitamins and minerals. It's also high in omega-3 fatty acids, which are beneficial to heart health. This recipe is a wonderful and healthful way to get your necessary amount of fish.

Poultry and meat

1. Lean beef and barley stew

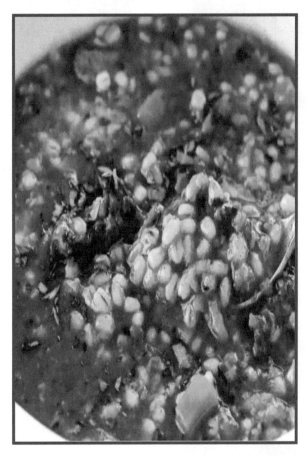

This delicious Lean Beef and Barley Stew is the ideal comfort dish on a chilly day. It contains lean protein, barley for healthy complex carbs, and a variety of veggies for a filling and enjoyable meal.

❖ **Preparation time:** 10 minutes
❖ **Cooking time:** 1 hour
❖ **Total time:** 1 hour 10 minutes

Ingredients:

❖ 1 tablespoon of olive oil.
❖ 1 pound of lean beef stew meat, trimmed and cut into 1 inch cubes
❖ 1 chopped onion
❖ 2 peeled and diced carrots.
❖ Two celery stalks, chopped
❖ 3 garlic cloves, minced
❖ 1 teaspoon dried thyme.
❖ 1/2 teaspoon dried rosemary.
❖ 1/2 teaspoon of salt.
❖ 1/4 teaspoon of black pepper.
❖ 4 cups beef broth
❖ 1 cup chopped tomatoes (fresh or tinned).
❖ 1 cup pearl barley, washed.
❖ 1 cup frozen peas.
❖ 1/4 cup freshly chopped parsley (optional)

Instructions:

❖ In a large Dutch oven or saucepan, warm the olive oil over medium heat. Add the steak and heat, tossing periodically, until browned on both sides.
❖ Cook the onion, carrots, and celery for 5 minutes, or until they are

softened. Stir in the garlic, thyme, rosemary, salt, and pepper.

❖ Pour in the beef broth and tomatoes. Bring to a boil, then decrease heat to low, cover, and let simmer for 45 minutes.

❖ Add the pearl barley and peas to the pot. Stir thoroughly, cover, and cook for another 30 minutes, or until the barley is soft and chewy.

❖ Remove from the fire and, if desired, add fresh parsley.

Serving Size: 6 Servings

Nutritional Information:

❖ **Calories:** Per serving: around 400
❖ **Carbohydrate:** 40 grams.
❖ **Fat:** 15 g
❖ **Protein:** 30 g
❖ **Vitamin A:** 20% Daily Value (DV).
❖ **Vitamin C:** 30%. DV
❖ **Fiber:** 5 g.

Cooking Tips:

❖ To make a thicker stew, use 1 tablespoon cornstarch with 2 tablespoons of water to form a slurry.

Stir the slurry into the stew for the final 5 minutes of simmering.

❖ You may substitute ground beef for stew meat. Simply brown the ground beef in the saucepan prior to adding the veggies.

❖ You may add extra veggies to this stew, such as potatoes, green beans, or mushrooms.

Health Benefits:

❖ Lean meat has plenty of protein and iron.

❖ Barley is a complete grain rich in fiber and complex carbs that can make you feel full and pleased.

❖ Vegetables are loaded with vitamins, minerals, and antioxidants.

❖ This stew is a substantial and healthy dinner that is ideal on a cold winter day.

2. Turkey and Spinach Stuffed Peppers

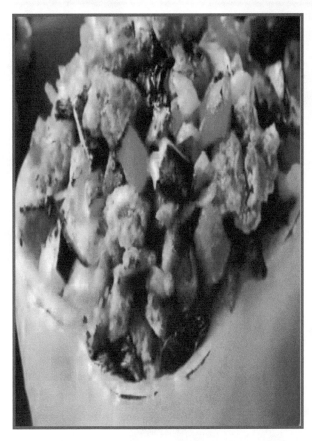

This dish turns bell peppers into edible bowls packed with flavorful ground turkey, rice, and spinach. Feel free to add your favorite veggies, such as sliced zucchini, mushrooms, or chopped onions.

- ❖ **Preparation time:** 15 minutes
- ❖ **Cooking time:** 40 minutes
- ❖ **Total time:** 55 minutes

Ingredients:

- ❖ 4 huge bell peppers, any color.

- ❖ 1 tablespoon of olive oil.
- ❖ 1 pound ground turkey
- ❖ 1/2 cup minced onion.
- ❖ 2 garlic cloves, minced
- ❖ 1 teaspoon of dried oregano.
- ❖ Add ½ teaspoon salt and ¼ teaspoon black pepper.
- ❖ 1 (14.5-ounce) can of chopped tomatoes, undrained
- ❖ 1/2 cup cooked brown rice.
- ❖ 5 ounces of chopped baby spinach
- ❖ 1/2 cup of shredded mozzarella cheese.
- ❖ ¼ cup chopped fresh parsley (optional)

Instructions:

- ❖ Preheat the oven to 375° Fahrenheit (190° Celsius). Wash and dry the bell peppers. Cut off the tops and remove the seeds and membranes. Trim a tiny slice off the bottom of each pepper to ensure it stands erect.
- ❖ In a large skillet, heat olive oil over medium heat. Add the ground turkey and heat, breaking it up with a spoon, until browned. Drain any extra grease.
- ❖ Add the onion and garlic and simmer for approximately 3 minutes, or until

softened. Combine oregano, salt, and pepper.

- ❖ Add chopped tomatoes (with liquids) and cooked brown rice. Bring to a simmer, then cook for 5 minutes.

- ❖ Add the chopped spinach and simmer for about 1 minute, or until wilted. Remove from heat.

- ❖ Divide the contents evenly between the prepped bell peppers. Place the peppers upright in a baking dish.

- ❖ Bake for 35-40 minutes, or until the peppers are soft and the filling is well cooked.

- ❖ Sprinkle mozzarella cheese on top of the peppers. Bake for a further 5 minutes, or until the cheese melts and bubbles.

- ❖ Garnish with fresh parsley (optional), and serve immediately.

Serving Size: 1 stuffed pepper.

Nutrition Facts: (per serving)

- ❖ **Calories:** 400.
- ❖ **Carbohydrates:** 35g
- ❖ **Fat:** 15g.
- ❖ **Protein:** 30 grams.
- ❖ **Vitamin A:** 30% of the Daily Value
- ❖ **Vitamin C:** 40%. DV

- ❖ **Fiber:** 4 grams.

Cooking Tips:

- ❖ When frying the ground turkey, add a sprinkle of red pepper flakes to make it spicier.

- ❖ Refrigerate leftovers in an airtight jar for up to three days. Reheat gently in an oven or microwave.

- ❖ To pre-cook the brown rice, follow the package directions and substitute 1/2 cup cooked rice into the recipe.

Health Benefits:

- ❖ This dish has a large amount of lean protein from ground turkey, which aids in muscle mass development and maintenance.

- ❖ Spinach contains a variety of vitamins and minerals, including vitamins A and C, which are essential for immune function and general health.

- ❖ Bell peppers provide vitamin C and fiber, both of which improve digestion.

3. Herb-Roasted Chicken and Vegetables

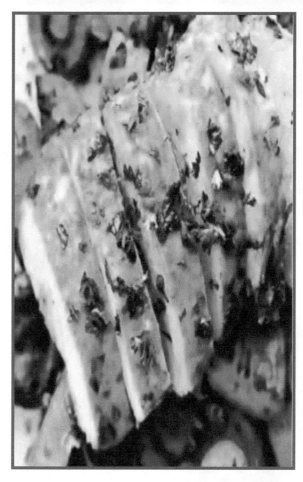

This one-pan marvel is an excellent evening supper! Tender, tasty chicken roasts with a cornucopia of bright veggies, all seasoned with a fragrant herb blend. It's a comprehensive and enjoyable meal that is simple to clean up after.

- ❖ **Preparation time:** 15 minutes
- ❖ **Cooking time:** 1 hour
- ❖ **Total time:** 1 hour and 15 minutes

Ingredients:

- ❖ 1 entire chicken (3 1/2 to 4 pounds), washed and patted dry.
- ❖ 2 tablespoons of olive oil.
- ❖ 1 tablespoon of chopped fresh rosemary
- ❖ 1 tablespoon of chopped fresh thyme.
- ❖ 1 teaspoon of dried oregano.
- ❖ 1/2 teaspoon paprika.
- ❖ 1/2 teaspoon of garlic powder.
- ❖ 1/2 teaspoon of onion powder.
- ❖ Add salt and freshly ground black pepper to taste.
- ❖ 3 medium potatoes, peeled and sliced into wedges
- ❖ 2 carrots, peeled and sliced into pieces
- ❖ 1 red onion sliced into wedges.
- ❖ 1 cup trimmed and halved Brussels sprouts.
- ❖ 1 lemon, sliced into wedges

Instructions:

- ❖ Preheat the oven to 425° Fahrenheit (220° Celsius).
- ❖ In a small mixing bowl, combine olive oil, rosemary, thyme, oregano,

paprika, garlic powder, onion powder, salt, and pepper.

- ❖ Rub the herb mixture all over the chicken, including beneath the skin. Season the cavities with salt and pepper.
- ❖ Put the chicken in a roasting pan. Spread the potatoes, carrots, onion, and Brussels sprouts around the chicken. Place the lemon slices into the cavity.
- ❖ Roast for 1 hour, or until the chicken is golden brown and fully cooked (165°F in the thickest part of the thigh). Baste the chicken and veggies with pan drippings halfway through roasting.

Serving Size: 4 servings

Nutritional Information: (Per Serving)

- ❖ **Calories:** 500
- ❖ **Carbohydrates:** 40g
- ❖ **Fat:** 30g
- ❖ **Protein:** 40g.
- ❖ **Vitamin C:** 10 percent DV
- ❖ **Fiber:** 5 grams.

Cooking Tips:

- ❖ Allow the chicken to lie uncovered at room temperature for 30 minutes before roasting to get extra crispy skin.
- ❖ If the veggies begin to brown too rapidly, tent the skillet with aluminum foil.
- ❖ To add a touch of sweetness, sprinkle the veggies with honey or maple syrup before roasting.

Health Benefits:

- ❖ Chicken contains a high concentration of lean protein, which is essential for muscle growth and maintenance.
- ❖ Vegetables include important vitamins, minerals, and fiber.
- ❖ Herbs like rosemary and thyme are anti-inflammatory.

Vegetarian Delights

1. Chickpea & Spinach Stew

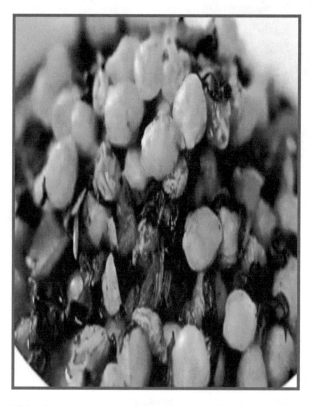

This hearty chickpea and spinach stew is a tasty and healthy one-pot dinner ideal for a busy weekday. It has protein and fiber from chickpeas, vitamins and minerals from spinach, and the pleasant aromas of your favorite spices. It's also simple to personalize using your preferred veggies and herbs.

- ❖ **Preparation time:** 10 minutes
- ❖ **Cook time:** 30 minutes
- ❖ **Total time:** 40 minutes

Ingredients:

- ❖ 1 tablespoon of olive oil.
- ❖ 1 medium onion, chopped.
- ❖ 2 garlic cloves, minced
- ❖ 1 teaspoon ground cumin.
- ❖ 1/2 teaspoon of smoked paprika.
- ❖ 1/4 teaspoon of red pepper flakes (optional)
- ❖ 1 (14.5-ounce) can of chopped tomatoes, undrained.
- ❖ 1 (15-ounce) can of chickpeas, washed and drained
- ❖ 4 cups veggie broth.
- ❖ 5 cups of baby spinach.
- ❖ Add salt and freshly ground black pepper to taste.
- ❖ 1/4 cup freshly chopped parsley (optional)

Instructions:

- ❖ In a big saucepan or Dutch oven, bring the olive oil to a medium heat. Cook until the onion softens, which should take around 5 minutes. Cook for a further 30 seconds after adding the garlic, cumin, paprika, and red pepper flakes (if used).
- ❖ Add chopped tomatoes with juices, chickpeas, and vegetable broth.

Bring to a boil, then decrease the heat and simmer for 15 minutes.

❖ Add the spinach and simmer for about 2 minutes, or until wilted. Season with salt and pepper to taste.

❖ Garnish with fresh parsley (if desired) and serve hot.

Serving Size: 4 servings

Nutritional Information:

- **Calories:** per serving (about 320).
- **Carbohydrate:** 40 grams.
- **Fat:** 10 grams.
- **Protein:** 15 g.
- **Vitamin A:** 20% of the Daily Value
- **Vitamin C:** 50% of the Daily Value
- **Fiber:** 8 g.

Cooking Tips:

❖ To make the stew thicker, mash some of the chickpeas against the pot's edge with a fork before adding the spinach.

❖ You may add other veggies to this stew, such as sliced carrots, bell peppers, or zucchini.

❖ If fresh spinach is not available, use 10 ounces of frozen spinach that has been thawed and drained.

❖ To make this stew vegan, leave off the parmesan cheese.

Health Benefits:

❖ This chickpea and spinach stew has plenty of plant-based protein and fiber, which will keep you full and content. It's also high in vitamins and minerals, like vitamin A, C, and iron. Spinach is an excellent source of folate, which is essential for pregnant women and those trying to conceive.

2. Lentil and Sweet Potato Curry

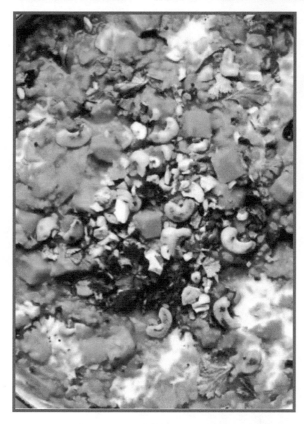

This aromatic curry is an excellent illustration of how simple ingredients may combine to provide a tasty and enjoyable dinner. The mix of sweet potatoes and lentils creates an excellent textural contrast, while the warming spices give depth and richness. It's an excellent recipe to prepare ahead of time for meal prep, and it stores nicely.

- ❖ **Preparation time:** 10 minutes
- ❖ **Cook time:** 30 minutes
- ❖ **Total time:** 40 minutes

Ingredients:

- ❖ 1 tablespoon of coconut oil.
- ❖ 1/2 medium onion, diced.
- ❖ 1 tablespoon of grated ginger.
- ❖ 3 garlic cloves, minced
- ❖ 1 teaspoon of curry powder.
- ❖ 1/2 teaspoon turmeric.
- ❖ 1/2 teaspoon of ground cumin
- ❖ 1/4 teaspoon of chili powder (optional)
- ❖ 1 (14.5-ounce) can of chopped tomatoes, undrained.
- ❖ 1 cup veggie broth.
- ❖ 1 cup red lentils, washed.
- ❖ 2 medium sweet potatoes, peeled and chopped
- ❖ 1 (13.5-ounce) can of light coconut milk.
- ❖ 1 tablespoon of chopped fresh cilantro.
- ❖ Add salt and freshly ground black pepper to taste.

Instructions:

- ❖ Heat the coconut oil in a big saucepan or Dutch oven over medium heat. Cook for 5 minutes, or until the onion has softened. Add the ginger, garlic, curry powder, turmeric, cumin, and chili powder (if using) and simmer for another minute, or until aromatic.

❖ Combine the diced tomatoes, vegetable broth, lentils, and sweet potatoes. Bring to a boil, then lower the heat, cover, and simmer for 20-25 minutes, or until the lentils and sweet potatoes are cooked.

❖ Stir in the coconut milk and cilantro. Season with salt and pepper to taste.

❖ Serve hot with rice or quinoa.

Serving size: Each dish yields four servings.

Nutritional Information:

❖ **Calories:** per serving (about 380).
❖ **Carbohydrates:** 45 grams.
❖ **Fat:** 15 g.
❖ **Protein:** 18 g.
❖ **Vitamin A:** 30% of the Daily Value
❖ **Fiber:** 8 g.

Cooking Tips:

❖ For a richer curry, mash some of the cooked sweet potatoes with a fork before adding the coconut milk.

❖ You may use any variety of lentil in this recipe, although red lentils cook the quickest. Brown or green lentils will also work, though they may take longer to cook.

❖ To make this meal vegan, substitute coconut milk and vegetable broth.

❖ This curry is also ideal for using up leftover cooked lentils or sweet potatoes.

Health Benefits:

❖ Lentils contain plant-based protein and fiber, which can make you feel full and pleased. They are also rich in iron, folate, and potassium.

❖ Sweet potatoes are rich in vitamins A and C, as well as fiber.

❖ This curry has high levels of antioxidants, which can help protect your cells from harm.

❖ The ingredients in this curry may also provide some health advantages. Turmeric, for example, has potent anti-inflammatory properties.

3. Stuffed Portobello Mushroom

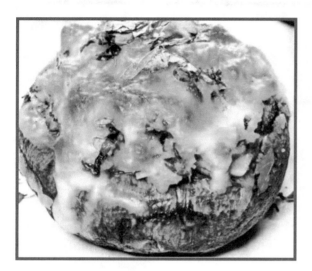

Stuffed portobello mushrooms are a tasty and filling vegetarian meal that can be served as a main course or as a side. Portobello mushrooms are huge, meaty mushrooms with a pleasant flavor and texture. When stuffed with a tasty filling, they provide a fulfilling and healthy meal.

This dish is an excellent way to savor portobello mushrooms. The mushrooms are packed with pork, veggies, and herbs before baking until soft and fragrant. You may tailor the filling to your preferences by adding different types of sausage, veggies, and cheese.

- ❖ **Preparation time:** 10 minutes
- ❖ **Cooking time:** 20 minutes
- ❖ **Total time:** 30 minutes

Ingredients:

- ❖ 4 huge Portobello mushrooms
- ❖ 1 tablespoon of olive oil.
- ❖ 1/2 medium onion, chopped.
- ❖ 1 clove garlic, minced
- ❖ 4 ounces of ground Italian sausage (or vegetarian sausage).
- ❖ 1/2 cup chopped spinach.
- ❖ 1/4 cup of chopped sun-dried tomatoes.
- ❖ 1/4 cup crumbled feta cheese.
- ❖ 1/4 cup shredded mozzarella cheese.
- ❖ 1/4 teaspoon of dried oregano.
- ❖ 1/4 teaspoon of dried thyme.
- ❖ Add salt and pepper to taste.

Instructions:

- ❖ Preheat the oven to 400° F (200° C). Line a baking sheet with parchment paper.
- ❖ Prepare the mushrooms by carefully removing the stems from the portobello mushrooms. Brush the mushrooms' tops and bottoms with olive oil. Season with salt and pepper. Place the mushrooms, gills facing up, on the prepared baking sheet.

- To prepare the filling, heat olive oil in a large pan over medium heat. Cook the onion and garlic for approximately 5 minutes, or until softened. Cook the sausage until browned, breaking it up with a spoon as it cooks.
- Combine the spinach, sun-dried tomatoes, feta cheese, oregano, and thyme. Cook for a few minutes until the spinach has wilted. Season with salt and pepper to taste.
- Stuff the mushrooms: Divide the filling evenly between the portobello mushrooms. Top with mozzarella cheese.
- Bake for 20 to 25 minutes, or until the mushrooms are soft and the cheese is melted and bubbling.
- Serve immediately.

Serving size: one filled portobello mushroom.

Nutrition Facts: (per serving)

- **Calories:** 350.
- **Carbohydrate:** 20 grams
- **Fat:** 20 g
- **Protein:** 25 grams
- **Vitamin C:** 2% DV
- **Fiber:** 3 grams

Cooking Tips:

- If you don't have fresh spinach, you may substitute frozen spinach. Thaw the spinach and squeeze away any extra moisture before mixing it into the filling.
- This dish may also be made with different varieties of cheese, such as ricotta, goat, or Parmesan.
- To make this dish vegan, substitute vegan sausage and leave off the feta cheese.

Health Benefits:

- Stuffed Portobello mushrooms are high in protein, fiber, and vitamins. They are low in calories and fat.
- Portobello mushrooms are rich in antioxidants, which can help protect your cells from harm.
- Sausage provides protein and iron to the meal.
- Spinach is rich in vitamins A, C, and K.
- Sun-dried tomatoes contain lycopene, an antioxidant associated with a variety of health advantages.

Chapter 7

Side Dish Recipes

Whole grains and legumes

1. Barley and Mushroom Risotto

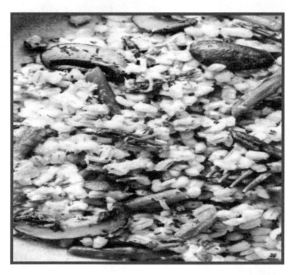

This Barley and Mushroom Risotto is a robust and savory take on the classic risotto, full of minerals and earthy richness. The barley provides a lovely chewy texture, while the mushrooms give a delicious depth. Ideal for a warm vegetarian supper.

- ❖ **Preparation time:** 10 minutes
- ❖ **Cooking time:** 45 minutes
- ❖ **Total time:** 55 minutes

Ingredients:

- ❖ 1 tablespoon of olive oil.
- ❖ 1 small onion, chopped.
- ❖ 2 garlic cloves, minced
- ❖ 1/2 cup dry white wine (optional)
- ❖ 8 ounces of assorted mushrooms, cleaned and sliced (cremini, white, portobello, or your preference)
- ❖ 3–4 cups of chicken or veggie broth
- ❖ 1 cup pearl barley.
- ❖ 1 tablespoon of fresh parsley, chopped
- ❖ ¼ cup finely shredded Parmesan cheese
- ❖ 1/2 tablespoon truffle oil (optional)
- ❖ Add salt and pepper to taste.

Instructions:

- ❖ Heat the olive oil in a large pot or Dutch oven over medium heat. Add the onion and simmer for 4 minutes, or until softened.

- Cook for a further 5 minutes, stirring periodically, after adding the mushrooms and garlic.
- Cook the barley for 2 minutes, stirring regularly.
- Pour in the white wine (if using) and heat until it has evaporated, scraping off any browned parts from the pan.
- Bring 3 cups of broth to a boil. Reduce the heat, cover, and simmer for 30 minutes, stirring periodically.
- If the liquid evaporates before the barley is cooked, add the remaining broth ½ cup at a time until the barley is soft, chewy, and has a slight bite (al dente). This may take another 15 minutes.
- Once cooked, remove from the pan and add half of the parmesan cheese, parsley, salt, and pepper to taste.
- Top with the remaining cheese and truffle oil (if using), then serve immediately.

Serving Size: Four servings

Nutritional Information (per Serving)

- **Calories:** 400.
- **Carbohydrate:** 50 grams
- **Fat:** 10g
- **Protein:** 15 grams.
- **Vitamin D:** 10% of the Daily Value
- **Fiber:** 5 grams.

Cooking Tips:

- For a fuller taste, use vegetable stock for chicken broth and sauté the onion and mushrooms with a tablespoon of butter.
- Toasted pearl barley provides a pleasant nutty richness. Toast the barley in a dry skillet over medium heat for 5 minutes before transferring it to the saucepan.
- If you do not have truffle oil, a drizzle of high-quality olive oil will suffice.
- Refrigerate leftovers in an airtight jar for up to three days. Reheat gently on the burner, adding a splash of broth as required to soften the texture.

Health Benefits:

- Barley is a complete grain high in fiber, which can aid digestion and increase feelings of fullness.
- Mushrooms are rich in antioxidants and vitamins, including vitamin D.

2. Brown Rice and Black Bean Salad

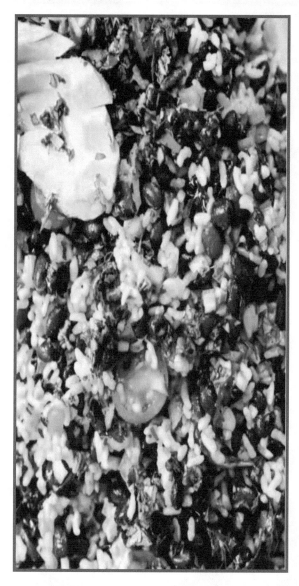

This vivid and fragrant Brown Rice and Black Bean Salad is a protein-packed vegetarian dish ideal for a light lunch, a refreshing side dish, or a filling main course. It's easy to personalize with your favorite add-ins, making it an excellent way to clean out the fridge.

❖ **Preparation time:** 10 minutes
❖ **Cooking Time:** 45 minutes (brown rice)
❖ **Total time:** 55 minutes

Ingredients:

❖ 1 ½ cup uncooked brown rice.
❖ 3 cups of water.
❖ 1 tablespoon of olive oil.
❖ ½ teaspoon salt.
❖ One (15-ounce) can of black beans, washed and drained
❖ 1 (15-ounce) canned corn, drained
❖ 1 (15.25-ounce) can of chopped tomatoes, undrained.
❖ 1/2 cup chopped red onion.
❖ 1/4 cup chopped fresh cilantro.
❖ 1 tablespoon of lime juice.
❖ 1 avocado sliced (optional)

Instructions:

❖ Cook the brown rice according to the package instructions. In a saucepan, mix together the brown rice, water, olive oil, and salt. Bring to a boil, then decrease heat, cover, and simmer for 45 minutes, or until the rice is cooked and the liquid has been absorbed. Remove from the heat and fluff with a fork. Allow to cool slightly.

- ❖ In a large mixing dish, add cooked brown rice, black beans, corn, chopped tomatoes, red onion, and cilantro.
- ❖ In a small bowl, combine the lime juice and olive oil. Toss the salad with the dressing until well coated.
- ❖ Serve immediately or refrigerate for up to three days. If desired, garnish with avocado slices before serving.

Serving Size: 6 Servings

Nutritional Information (per Serving)

- ❖ **Calories:** 300.
- ❖ **Carbohydrate:** 45g
- ❖ **Fat:** 8g
- ❖ **Protein:** 12 grams.
- ❖ **Vitamin A:** 20% of the Daily Value
- ❖ **Fiber:** 5 grams.

Cooking Tips:

- ❖ Cook the brown rice in vegetable broth rather than water for a more flavorful result.
- ❖ Chopped bell pepper, cucumber, or jalapeño can be used to enhance flavor and texture.
- ❖ Leftovers can be served cold or gently warmed in a pan or microwave.

Health Benefits:

- ❖ Brown rice is a complete grain high in fiber, which aids digestion and keeps you feeling fuller for longer. Black beans are an excellent source of plant-based protein and iron. This salad is also rich in vitamins and minerals, such as vitamin A and fiber.

3. Quinoa Pilaf With Herbs

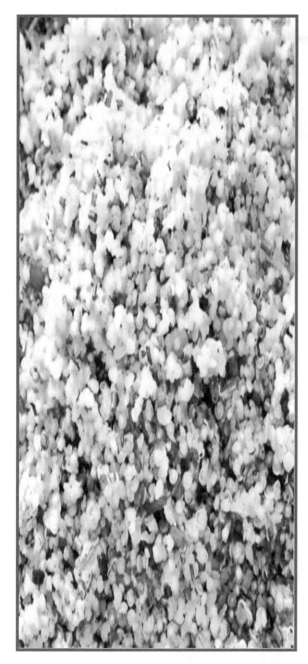

Quinoa pilaf is a delicious and nutritious side dish cooked with quinoa, a complete protein grain, and fresh herbs. It's an excellent complement to roasted chicken, grilled seafood, or vegetarian meals.

❖ **Preparation time:** 5 minutes
❖ **Cooking time:** 20 minutes
❖ **Total time:** 25 minutes

Ingredients:

❖ 1 cup of quinoa, rinsed
❖ 1 1/2 cups chicken or veggie broth
❖ 1 tablespoon of olive oil.
❖ 1/2 cup diced onion
❖ 1/4 cup chopped fresh parsley.
❖ 2 tablespoons of chopped fresh cilantro.
❖ 1 teaspoon dried thyme.
❖ 1/2 teaspoon of salt.
❖ 1/4 teaspoon of black pepper.
❖ 1/4 cup chopped walnuts or pecans (optional).

Instructions:

❖ In a saucepan, heat the olive oil over medium heat. Cook until the onion softens, which should take around 5 minutes.
❖ Stir in the rinsed quinoa and simmer for 1 minute, stirring regularly.
❖ Combine broth, thyme, salt, and pepper. Bring to a boil, then decrease the heat, cover, and cook for 15

minutes, or until the quinoa is fluffy and the liquid has been absorbed.

❖ Remove from the heat and fluff with a fork. Mix in the parsley, cilantro, and walnuts (if using).

❖ Serve warm.

Serving size: Each dish yields four servings.

Nutrition Information:

❖ **Calories per serving:** 220

❖ **Carbohydrate:** 35 grams per serving

❖ **Fat:** 8 grams

❖ **Protein:** 8 grams

❖ **Fiber:** 4 grams

❖ **Vitamin A:** 10% daily value (DV)

❖ **Iron:** 15% DV.

Cooking Tips:

❖ To enhance the flavor, toast the quinoa in the olive oil before adding the broth.

❖ You may use any broth instead of the vegetable or chicken broth.

❖ Add additional chopped veggies to the pilaf, such as bell peppers, carrots, and zucchini.

❖ To make the meal vegan, eliminate the walnuts and pecans.

Health Benefits:

❖ Quinoa pilaf is a healthy and tasty side dish. Quinoa provides protein, fiber, and all nine essential amino acids. This meal is also rich in vitamins and minerals, such as iron and vitamin A.

Vegetable Sides

1. Garlic Sautéed Spinach

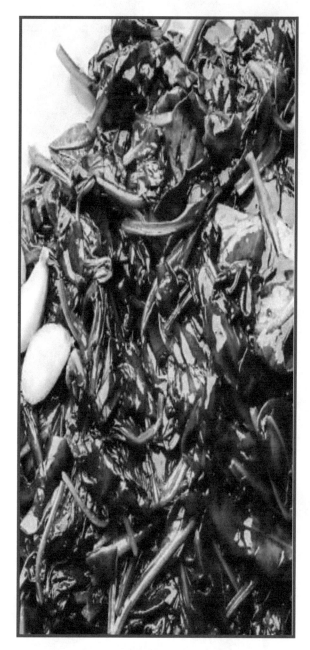

Garlic Sautéed Spinach is a simple yet nutritious side dish. It pairs well with any protein and may also be consumed on its own as a light meal.

❖ **Preparation time:** 5 minutes
❖ **Cooking time:** 5 minutes
❖ **Total time:** 10 minutes

Ingredients:

❖ 2 bunches of fresh spinach (or a 10-ounce package)
❖ 1 tablespoon of olive oil.
❖ 2 garlic cloves, minced
❖ Add salt and pepper to taste (optional). Add 1 squeeze of lemon juice (optional). A pinch of red pepper flakes.

Instructions:

❖ Wash the spinach well with cold water. Remove any stiff stems.
❖ Heat olive oil in a large skillet or pan over medium heat. Add the minced garlic and heat for 30 seconds, or until fragrant but not browned.
❖ Cook the spinach, stirring regularly, until wilted, about 2-3 minutes. The spinach will shrivel significantly as it wilts.
❖ Season with salt and pepper to taste. Remove from the heat and, if preferred, add a squeeze of lemon juice.

❖ Serve immediately.

Serving size per recipe: 2 servings.

Nutrition Facts: (per serving)

- ❖ **Calories:** 41
- ❖ **Carbohydrate:** 4 grams
- ❖ **Fat:** 3 g
- ❖ **Protein:** 2 grams
- ❖ **Vitamin A:** 25% of the Daily Value
- ❖ **Vitamin C:** 15 percent DV
- ❖ **Fiber:** 1 g

Cooking Tips:

- ❖ Do not overcook the spinach! If cooked for an extended period of time, it will rapidly wilt and turn to pulp.
- ❖ You may use any oil you prefer, including avocado oil, grapeseed oil, and butter.
- ❖ Add a pinch of red pepper flakes for some spice.
- ❖ To save time, pre-wash and cut the spinach.

Health Benefits:

- ❖ Spinach has high levels of vitamins A and C, as well as fiber.
- ❖ It's also rich in iron, folate, and potassium.
- ❖ Garlic is well-known for its immune-boosting properties and ability to reduce inflammation.

2. Steamed asparagus with lemon

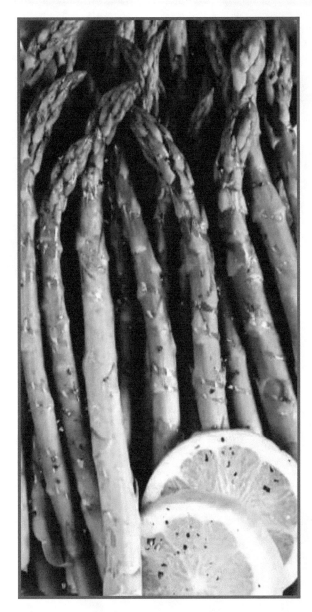

This recipe for steamed asparagus with lemon exemplifies how minimal preparation can provide a tasty and nutritious side dish. With only a few ingredients and little prep work, you can have excellent asparagus on the table in under 10 minutes.

❖ **Preparation time:** 5 minutes

❖ **Cooking time:** 4–5 minutes

❖ **Total time:** 9-10 minutes

Ingredients:

❖ 1 bunch fresh asparagus (about 12-15 spears)

❖ 1 tablespoon of unsalted butter.

❖ 1 lemon.

❖ Add ½ teaspoon salt and ¼ teaspoon freshly ground black pepper.

Instructions:

❖ Wash the asparagus well and cut the woody ends. Simply snap off the asparagus ends where they naturally break.

❖ Fill a saucepan with approximately 1 inch of water. Bring the water to a boil over medium heat.

❖ While the water heats, melt the butter in a small bowl. Squeeze half of the lemon and add it to the melted butter. Season with salt and pepper.

❖ Place the steamer basket in the boiling water. Place the asparagus in the steamer basket and cover the pot.

❖ Steam asparagus for 4-5 minutes, or until soft and crisp. The asparagus should be bright green with a tiny sharpness.

- ❖ Remove the asparagus from the steamer basket and place it on a serving platter.
- ❖ Drizzle the asparagus with the lemon butter sauce and serve immediately.

Serving Size: This dish makes 2-3 servings.

Nutritional Information (per Serving)

- ❖ **Calories:** 40.
- ❖ **Carbohydrate:** 5 grams
- ❖ **Fat:** 3 g.
- ❖ **Protein:** 2 grams.
- ❖ **Vitamin C:** 25% DV
- ❖ **Fiber:** 1 gram.

Cooking Tips:

- ❖ For thicker asparagus spears, steam them for an extra minute or two.
- ❖ If you do not have a steamer basket, use a colander that fits tightly over the top of the pot.
- ❖ You may use olive oil instead of butter to have a deeper taste.
- ❖ To add a hint of garlic, mince a tiny clove and mix it into the melted butter.

Health Benefits:

- ❖ Asparagus is a nutritionally dense, low-calorie vegetable. It is rich in vitamins A, C, K, and folate. Asparagus contains fiber, which aids digestion and promotes feelings of fullness.

3.   Roasted   Brussels sprouts with Almonds

❖ **Preparation time:** 10 minutes

❖ **Cooking time:** 25-30 minutes

❖ **Total Time:** 35-40 minutes

Ingredients:

❖ 1 pound of Brussels sprouts, cut and halved

❖ 2 tablespoons olive oil

❖ 1/2 teaspoon salt

❖ 1/4 teaspoon black pepper.

❖ 1/2 cup sliced almonds.

❖ 1 tablespoon of fresh lemon juice (optional).

Instructions:

❖ Preheat the oven to 400° F (200° C). Line a baking sheet with parchment paper.

❖ In a large dish, toss the Brussels sprouts with olive oil, salt, and pepper. Spread the Brussels sprouts in a single layer on the prepared baking sheet.

❖ Roast for 20-25 minutes, or until the Brussels sprouts are soft and golden brown, tossing halfway through.

❖ While the Brussels sprouts roast, toast the almonds in a dry pan over medium heat until golden brown,

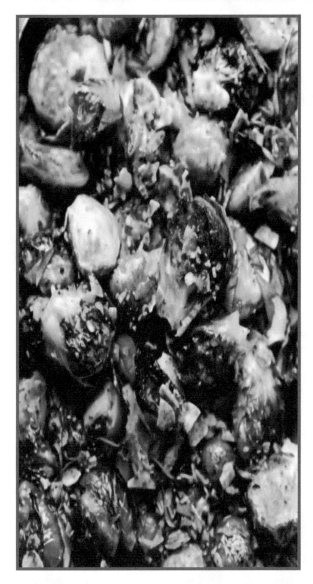

Roasted Brussels sprouts are a simple and tasty side dish that can be eaten throughout the year. Brussels sprouts have a somewhat nutty taste that goes well with the crunch of roasted almonds. This dish is simple to follow and needs little preparation time, making it an excellent weeknight alternative.

turning regularly. Take care not to toast the almonds.

- ❖ When the Brussels sprouts are done, take them from the oven and combine with the toasted almonds.
- ❖ Serve immediately with a squeeze of fresh lemon juice, if desired.

Serving size: This recipe yields around four servings.

Nutrition Facts: (per serving)

- ❖ **Calories:** 150.
- ❖ **Carbohydrates:** 15g
- ❖ **Fat:** 9g.
- ❖ **Protein:** 5 grams.
- ❖ **Vitamin C:** 70%. DV
- ❖ **Fiber:** 3 grams.

Cooking Tips:

- ❖ Cut Brussels sprouts into tiny wedges rather than half for additional crispy results.
- ❖ If you don't have fresh lemon juice, you may use 1 teaspoon balsamic vinegar.
- ❖ To add a touch of sweetness, sprinkle the roasted Brussels sprouts with a spoonful of maple syrup or honey before serving.

Health Benefits:

- ❖ Brussels sprouts are rich in vitamins C and K, as well as fiber.
- ❖ Almonds include nutritious fats, protein, and fiber.
- ❖ This recipe is a low-calorie, low-carb side dish that compliments a nutritious supper

Chapter 8

Fruit-Based Desserts Recipes

1. Banana & Walnut Bread

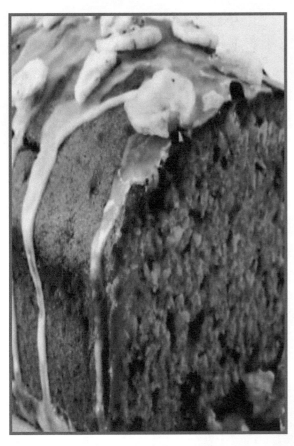

This tasty and moist banana walnut bread is a great teatime treat or healthy snack. It's a terrific way to use up overripe bananas and will undoubtedly become a favorite!

- ❖ **Preparation time:** 10 minutes
- ❖ **Cooking time:** 50-60 minutes
- ❖ **Total time:** 1 hour

Ingredients:

- ❖ 3 very ripe bananas, mashed (approximately 1 1/3 cups).
- ❖ 1/2 cup (1 stick) unsalted butter, softened
- ❖ 3/4 cup granulated sugar.
- ❖ 2 big eggs, lightly beaten
- ❖ 1 1/2 cups all-purpose flour.
- ❖ 1 teaspoon of baking soda.
- ❖ 1/2 teaspoon salt
- ❖ 1 teaspoon vanilla essence.
- ❖ 1 cup chopped walnuts.

Instructions:

- ❖ Preheat the oven to 350°F (175°C). Grease and flour a loaf pan (8 x 4 inches).
- ❖ In a large mixing basin, beat together the softened butter and sugar until light and fluffy.
- ❖ Beat in the eggs one at a time, then add the vanilla extract.

- ❖ Add the mashed bananas and stir until thoroughly blended.
- ❖ In a separate basin, mix the flour, baking soda, and salt.
- ❖ Gradually add the dry ingredients to the wet components, stirring until just blended. Do not overmix!
- ❖ Gently fold in the chopped walnuts.
- ❖ Pour the batter into the prepared loaf pan.
- ❖ Bake for 50–60 minutes, or until a toothpick inserted in the center comes out clean.
- ❖ Allow the bread to sit in the pan for 10 minutes before transferring it to a wire rack to cool fully.

Cooking Tips:

- ❖ Brown sugar can be used instead of granulated sugar to make the bread more moist.
- ❖ If you don't have walnuts, you may use pecans, chopped almonds, or even chocolate chips.
- ❖ Ripen your bananas by leaving them in a brown paper bag with an apple for a day or two.
- ❖ To keep the bread from drying out, cover it securely in plastic wrap or place it in an airtight container.

Serving Size: 1 slice (about 1 inch thick)

Nutrition Facts: (per slice)

- ❖ **Calories:** 280
- ❖ **Carbohydrates: 38**
- ❖ **Fat:** 12 g
- ❖ **Protein:** 4 grams.
- ❖ **Vitamin A** (2% DV)
- ❖ **Vitamin C:** 2%. DV
- ❖ **Fiber:** 1 g.

2. Almond Flour Brownies

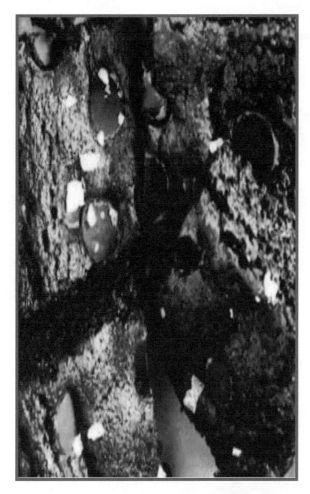

Ingredients:

- ❖ 1 1/2 cups almond flour.
- ❖ 1 teaspoon of baking powder.
- ❖ 1/2 teaspoon of salt.
- ❖ 5 tablespoons butter, melted and cooled somewhat.
- ❖ 1 3/4 cups granulated sweetener (erythritol, allulose, or coconut sugar)
- ❖ 3/4 cup unsweetened cocoa powder.
- ❖ Three big eggs at room temperature.
- ❖ 1 teaspoon of vanilla essence.
- ❖ 1/2 cup of chocolate chips (optional)

Indulge your sweet taste with these luscious Almond Flour Brownies, a tasty and gluten-free alternative to traditional brownies. These brownies, made with almond flour and natural sweeteners, are thick and fudgy, making them ideal for any occasion.

- ❖ **Preparation time:** 10 minutes
- ❖ **Cooking time:** 25 to 35 minutes
- ❖ **Total time:** 45 minutes

Instructions:

- ❖ Preheat the oven to 350°F/175°C and line an 8x8 inch baking tray with parchment paper.
- ❖ In a larger basin, combine the almond flour, baking powder, and salt. Set aside.
- ❖ In a large mixing basin, whisk together the melted butter, sweetener, and vanilla extract until smooth.
- ❖ Beat in the eggs one at a time, stirring well after each addition.
- ❖ Gradually add the dry ingredients to the wet components, stirring until

just blended. Take care not to overmix.

- ❖ If you are using chocolate chips, fold them in.
- ❖ Pour the batter into the prepared baking pan and distribute evenly.
- ❖ Bake for 25–35 minutes, or until a toothpick inserted into the middle yields a few moist crumbs.
- ❖ Allow the brownies to cool fully in their pan before cutting and serving.

Serving Size: This recipe makes around 16 brownies.

Nutrition facts (per brownie):

- ❖ **Calories:** 300–350 (depending on the sweetener used).
- ❖ **Carbohydrates:** 20-25 grams (depending on the sweetener chosen).
- ❖ **Fat:** 20g
- ❖ **Protein:** 5 grams.
- ❖ **Vitamin E:** 7 mg.
- ❖ **Fiber:** 2 grams.

Cooking Tips:

- ❖ Reduce the baking time for fudgier brownies. Bake for a few minutes longer to achieve a cakier texture.
- ❖ If your almond flour is exceptionally fine, you may need to use slightly less.
- ❖ To ensure perfect setting, allow the brownies to cool fully before cutting.
- ❖ To prepare these dairy-free brownies, substitute vegan butter or coconut oil.

Health Benefits:

- ❖ Almond flour contains healthful lipids, protein, and fiber.
- ❖ This dish is gluten-free, making it an excellent choice for folks who are gluten sensitive.
- ❖ Using natural sweeteners such as erythritol or allulose reduces the overall sugar level.

3. Dark chocolate avocado mousse

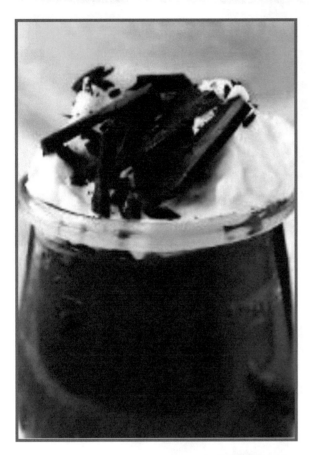

This luscious Dark Chocolate Avocado Mousse is a tasty and nutritious take on a traditional dessert. It's rich, creamy, and delicious, but it's also surprisingly healthy! This mousse, made with ripe avocados, dark chocolate, and a dash of maple syrup, is naturally sweet and high in healthy fats.

- ❖ **Preparation time:** 5 minutes
- ❖ **Cooking time:** 0 minutes
- ❖ **Total time:** 5 minutes

Ingredients:

- ❖ 2 ripe avocados.
- ❖ 4 ounces dark chocolate (70% cacao or more), melted
- ❖ ¼ cup unsweetened cocoa powder, ⅓ cup unsweetened almond milk, and ⅓ cup maple syrup.
- ❖ ½ teaspoon vanilla extract.
- ❖ ¼ teaspoon of ground cinnamon
- ❖ A pinch of sea salt.

Instructions:

- ❖ Combine all ingredients in a food processor or high-powered blender.
- ❖ Process until totally smooth and creamy, scraping down the sides as necessary.
- ❖ Place the mousse in serving plates and refrigerate for at least 1 hour, or until set.

Serving size: Each dish yields 4 servings.

Nutritional Information: (Approximated values per serving)

- ❖ **Calories:** 380
- ❖ **Carbs:** 30g
- ❖ **Fat:** 20g

- ❖ **Protein:** 4 grams
- ❖ **Vitamin C:** 2 mg
- ❖ **Fiber:** 7 grams

Cooking Tips:

- ❖ Melted chocolate chips can be used in place of baking chocolate to make a richer mousse.
- ❖ If the mixture is too thick, add a spoonful of almond milk at a time until the correct consistency is achieved.
- ❖ For the greatest texture, use avocados that are absolutely ripe. Unripe avocados will not mix well and have a grassy taste.

Health Benefits:

- ❖ Avocados include plenty of healthful fats, fiber, and vitamins.
- ❖ Dark chocolate is high in antioxidants and may benefit heart health.
- ❖ This mousse is a fantastic way to fulfill your sweet taste while avoiding the guilt!

4. Grilled Peaches with Greek Yogurt

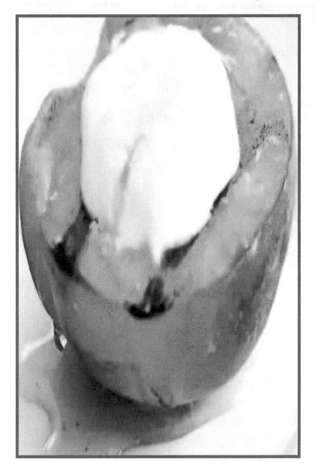

This is a simple and pleasant summer treat that takes only minutes to make. Grilled peaches have a smoky sweetness that goes well with the cold smoothness of Greek yogurt. It's a healthful and delectable dessert that may be eaten alone or with your favorite toppings.

- ❖ **Preparation time:** 5 minutes
- ❖ **Cooking time:** 8–10 minutes
- ❖ **Total time:** 13-15 minutes

Ingredients:

- ❖ 2 juicy peaches.
- ❖ 1/2 cup plain Greek yogurt.
- ❖ 1 tablespoon honey.
- ❖ 1/2 a teaspoon of crushed cinnamon
- ❖ A pinch of powdered nutmeg (optional).
- ❖ Fresh mint leaves for garnish (optional).

Instructions:

- ❖ Preheat the grill or grill pan to medium heat.
- ❖ Cut each peach in half and remove the pits.
- ❖ In a small dish, mix together the Greek yogurt, honey, cinnamon, and nutmeg (if using).
- ❖ (Optional) Lightly oil the cut sides of the peaches.
- ❖ Place the peaches, cut side down, on a grill or grill pan.
- ❖ Grill for 4-5 minutes on each side, or until soft and gently charred.
- ❖ Remove the peaches from the grill and spread the yogurt mixture in the center of each half.
- ❖ Garnish with fresh mint leaves if preferred.

Serving size: 1 peach half with yogurt topping.

Nutritional Information (per Serving)

- ❖ **Calories:** 180
- ❖ **Carbohydrate:** 25 grams
- ❖ **Fat:** 3g
- ❖ **Protein:** 8 grams
- ❖ **Vitamin C:** 6mg (4% of DV)
- ❖ **Fiber:** 2 grams

Cooking Tips:

- ❖ Vanilla-flavored Greek yogurt adds a deeper taste.
- ❖ If you don't have a grill, broil the peaches in the oven for a few minutes until tender and gently browned.
- ❖ To keep the peaches from sticking to the grill, gently oil them before cooking. This is unnecessary if your grill is clean and well-heated.

Health Benefits:

- ❖ Peaches include a variety of vitamins and minerals, including vitamin C and fiber.
- ❖ Greek yogurt is a good source of protein and calcium.
- ❖ This dessert is a healthier alternative to sweet foods while providing lots of satisfaction.

5. Berries with Oat Crisp

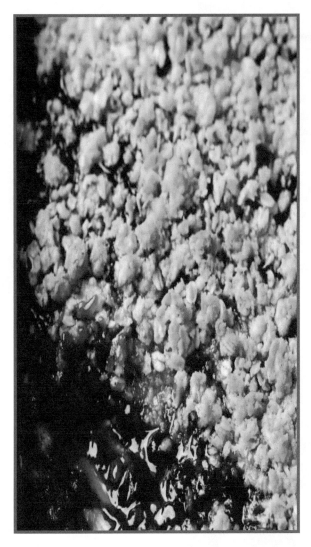

Berry & Oat Crisp is a delicious and easy dish filled with luscious berries and a satisfyingly crispy oat crumble topping. It's ideal for a summer potluck or a relaxing night in.

- ❖ **Preparation time:** 15 minutes
- ❖ **Cooking time:** 40 to 45 minutes
- ❖ **Total time:** 1 hour

Ingredients:

- ❖ To make the Crisp Topping, combine 1 ½ cups rolled oats.
- ❖ 1 cup all-purpose flour.
- ❖ 1/2 cup packed brown sugar.
- ❖ 1/4 cup granulated sugar.
- ❖ 1 teaspoon ground cinnamon.
- ❖ ½ teaspoon salt.
- ❖ 1/2 cup (1 stick) cold, unsalted butter, cubed

For the berry filling:

- ❖ 4 cups fresh or frozen mixed berries (strawberries, blueberries, raspberries, and blackberries)
- ❖ 3/4 cup granulated sugar
- ❖ 3 tablespoons cornstarch.
- ❖ 1 tablespoon of lemon juice.
- ❖ 1/2 teaspoon vanilla extract (optional)

Instructions:

- ❖ Preheat the oven to 375° Fahrenheit (190° Celsius). Grease an 8-by-8-inch baking dish.
- ❖ Make the crisp topping: In a large mixing basin, combine the oatmeal, flour, brown sugar, granulated sugar,

cinnamon, and salt. Cut in the chilled butter with a pastry cutter or your fingertips until the mixture is the consistency of coarse crumbs. Set aside.

❖ Make the berry filling: In another basin, mix together the berries, sugar, cornstarch, lemon juice, and vanilla extract (if using). Gently toss the berries to provide a uniform coating.

❖ Pour the berry filling into the prepared baking dish. Sprinkle the oat crumble topping evenly over the berries.

❖ Bake for 40-45 minutes, or until the filling bubbles and the topping turns golden brown.

❖ Allow to cool slightly before serving. Enjoy warm with vanilla ice cream, whipped cream, or by itself.

Serving Size: 8 servings

Nutritional Information (Per Serving):

❖ **Calories:** 350
❖ **Carbohydrate:** 50 grams
❖ **Fat:** 15g
❖ **Protein:** 4 grams
❖ **Vitamin C:** High (from berries)

❖ **Fiber:** 4 grams

Cooking Tips:

❖ Use brown butter in the crumble topping to give it a deeper taste. To brown butter, just melt it in a pot over medium heat, turning regularly, until golden brown and emitting a nutty scent.

❖ Do not overmix the crumble topping. A few bigger crumbles are ideal for adding texture.

❖ If your berries are really juicy, you may wish to add an extra tablespoon of cornstarch to the filling.

❖ To avoid a soggy bottom crust, preheat the baking dish before adding the berry filling.

Health Benefits:

❖ Berries contain high levels of antioxidants and vitamins, including vitamin C.

❖ Oatmeal contains fiber, which aids digestion and keeps you full.

6. Baked apples with cinnamon and nuts

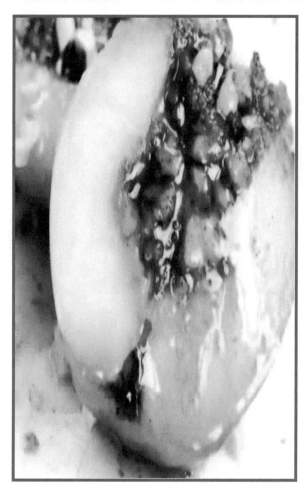

Baked apples are a nutritious and delicious dessert that is warm, soothing, and completely customizable. This recipe is basic with a classic combo of cinnamon and almonds, but feel free to be creative with your favorite ingredients!

- ❖ **Preparation time:** 10 minutes
- ❖ **Cooking time:** 45–50 minutes
- ❖ **Total Time:** 55-60 minutes

Ingredients:

- ❖ 4 medium apples (Gala, Granny Smith, or Honeycrisp)
- ❖ 1/4 cup chopped walnuts.
- ❖ 1/4 cup packed light brown sugar.
- ❖ 1 teaspoon ground cinnamon.
- ❖ 2 tablespoons of unsalted butter, melted
- ❖ 1/4 cup water.

Instructions:

- ❖ Preheat the oven to 375° Fahrenheit (190° Celsius). Lightly oil a baking dish.
- ❖ Wash and core the apples. Using a sharp knife, remove a circular core from the top of each apple, keeping the bottom intact. If you have a melon baller, you may utilize it at this stage.
- ❖ In a small bowl, mix together the chopped walnuts, brown sugar, and cinnamon.
- ❖ Fill the apple cavity with nut mixture. Drizzle each apple with melted butter.
- ❖ Pour the water into the bottom of the baking dish. This will assist to keep the apples from drying out.

- Bake for 45–50 minutes, or until the apples are soft and cooked through. When you press your finger against the apples, they will yield slightly.
- Allow the apples to cool slightly before serving. Serve warm, topped with a dollop of vanilla ice cream, whipped cream, or honey (optional).

Serving Size: 1 apple

Nutrition Facts: (per serving)

- **Calories:** 230
- **Carbohydrates:** 40g
- **Fat:** 5g
- **Protein:** 2 grams
- **Vitamin C:** 6mg (4% of DV).
- **Fiber:** 4 grams

Cooking Tips:

- For a softer apple, bake for the entire 50 minutes. If you want extra texture, bake for 45 minutes.
- You may use pecans, almonds, or pistachios instead of walnuts.
- To add a touch of sweetness, sprinkle the apples with a spoonful of honey or maple syrup before baking.

- For a more luxurious treat, load the apples with a variety of chopped dried fruit, such as raisins, cranberries, or dates, as well as nuts and spices.

Health Benefits:

- Baked apples are a naturally delicious and delightful treat that is also nutritionally beneficial. Apples are rich in fiber, vitamin C, and antioxidants. Nuts in this dish provide healthful fats, protein, and extra vitamins and minerals.

7. Baked pears with cinnamon and honey

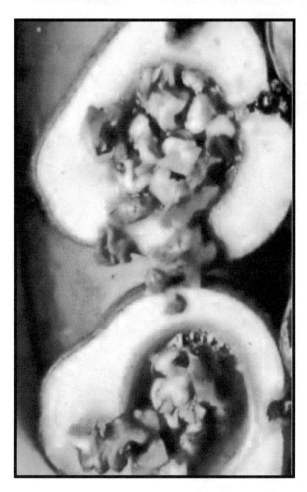

This simple and beautiful dish highlights the natural sweetness of pears. Baked pears are delicate, sensitive, and flavorful thanks to the heated cinnamon and drizzled honey. It's a nutritious and pleasant delicacy that may be eaten warm or cold.

- **Preparation time:** 10 minutes
- **Cooking Time:** 30–35 minutes
- **Total Time:** 40-45 minutes

Ingredients:

- ❖ 3 Bosc pears.
- ❖ 3/4 cup chopped walnuts (optional).
- ❖ 3 tablespoons of honey.
- ❖ Ground Cinnamon
- ❖ 1 tablespoon of water (optional)

Instructions:

- ❖ Preheat the oven to 350° Fahrenheit (175° Celsius).
- ❖ Wash the pears, then cut them in half lengthwise. Take a spoon and scoop out the core, leaving a little hollow in the middle.
- ❖ If using walnuts, chop them and place one teaspoon in the hollow of each pear half.
- ❖ Drizzle each pear half with about 1 teaspoon honey. Sprinkle liberally with ground cinnamon.
- ❖ To keep the pears from drying out, place them in a small baking dish with a tablespoon of water. Put the pear halves in the baking dish, cut side down.
- ❖ Bake for 30–35 minutes, or until the pears are soft and readily punctured with a fork.

- ❖ Allow the pears to cool slightly before serving. You may eat them heated or at room temperature.

Serving Size: 1 pear half.

Nutrition Facts: (per serving)

- ❖ **Calories:** 180
- ❖ **Carbohydrates:** 40g
- ❖ **Fat:** 3g.
- ❖ **Protein:** 1 g.
- ❖ **Vitamin C:** 8%. DV
- ❖ **Fiber:** 4 grams.

Cooking Tips:

- ❖ Brown sugar can be used in place of part of the honey to add a deeper taste.
- ❖ If your pears are not quite ripe, bake for an extra 5-10 minutes.
- ❖ To add a touch of luxury, garnish the cooked pears with whipped cream or vanilla ice cream.

Health Benefits:

- ❖ Pears include a high fiber content, which aids digestion and promotes feelings of fullness.
- ❖ Honey is a natural sweetener with antioxidants and antimicrobial properties.
- ❖ Cinnamon is a spice that has been demonstrated to help control blood sugar.

Chapter 9

Nutritious Smoothies and Beverages

1. Pomegranate and Green Tea Mocktail

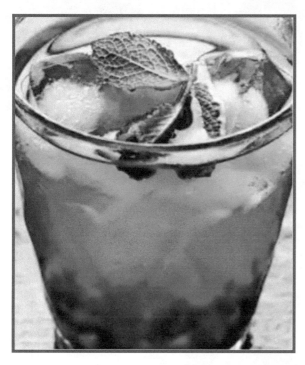

This refreshing mocktail mixes the slight bitterness of green tea with the sweet and tart flavor of pomegranate juice, resulting in a delicious and healthful drink. It's ideal for a hot summer day or when you need a pick-me-up without alcohol.

- ❖ **Preparation time:** 5 minutes
- ❖ **Cooking Time:** N/A
- ❖ **Total time:** 5 minutes

Ingredients:

- ❖ 1 cup brewed green tea, cooled.
- ❖ 1/2 cup of pomegranate juice.
- ❖ 1/4 cup club soda or sparkling water.
- ❖ 1 tablespoon honey (optional)
- ❖ 1/4 cup fresh pomegranate arils, or seeds.
- ❖ Fresh mint leaves for garnish (optional).

Instructions:

- ❖ In a pitcher or glass, combine the iced green tea with the pomegranate juice and honey (if using). Stir thoroughly.
- ❖ Gently mix in the club soda or sparkling water.
- ❖ Pour the mocktail into glasses with ice.
- ❖ Garnish with fresh pomegranate arils and mint leaves (optional).

Serving Size: 1 glass.

Nutritional Information: (Approximated values per serving)

- ❖ **Calories:** 50
- ❖ **Carbohydrate:** 12g
- ❖ **Fat:** 0g
- ❖ **Protein:** 1 g
- ❖ **Vitamin C:** 20 percent DV
- ❖ **Fiber:** 1 g

Cooking Tips:

- ❖ Replace the pomegranate juice with homemade grenadine for a richer pomegranate taste. To prepare grenadine, combine equal parts pomegranate juice and sugar and heat until the sugar dissolves and the liquid thickens slightly.
- ❖ If you don't have fresh pomegranate arils, you can use frozen arils (thawed) or another fruit, such as raspberries or cranberries.
- ❖ Instead of tea bags, use loose leaf tea to get a stronger green tea flavor. Steep the tea for 3-5 minutes, depending on your desired strength.

Health Benefits:

- ❖ Green tea has high levels of antioxidants, which can help protect your cells from harm.
- ❖ Pomegranate juice is abundant in antioxidants and has been proved to be anti-inflammatory.
- ❖ This mocktail is a healthier, more refreshing alternative to sugary drinks and juices.

2. Herbal-infused water

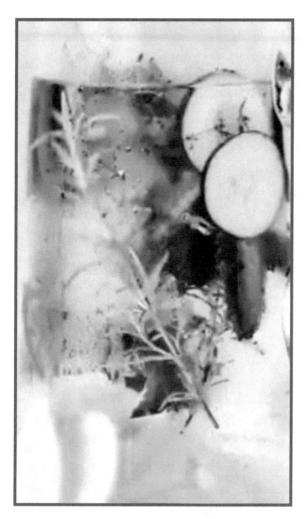

Herbal infused water is a delightful and healthful approach to replace sugary beverages and increase your water consumption. It's packed with flavor from the infused herbs and may be tailored to your liking. Plus, it's quite simple to create!

- ❖ **Preparation time:** 5 minutes
- ❖ **Cooking time:** 0 minutes
- ❖ **Total time:** 5 minutes

Ingredients:

- 4-6 sprigs of fresh herbs (mint, basil, rosemary, thyme, etc.).
- 1 liter of filtered water.
- Optional: sliced fruits (citrus fruits, berries, cucumber).

Instructions:

- ❖ Wash the herbs and fruits well. If you're using fruits, slice them thinly.
- ❖ Muddle the herbs gently to unleash their flavors.
- ❖ Place the herbs and fruits (if using) in a pitcher of filtered water.
- ❖ Cover the pitcher and chill for at least 4 hours, preferably overnight, for a stronger taste.
- ❖ Enjoy chilling!

Serving size: 1 Liter (4 Cups)

Nutritional Information:

- ❖ **Calories:** Nearly insignificant (mostly from fruits, if used).
- ❖ **Carbohydrates:** Nearly insignificant (mostly from fruits, if used).
- ❖ **Fat:** 0g
- ❖ **Protein:** 0 grams

- ❖ **Vitamin C:** Excellent source (when utilizing citrus fruits).
- ❖ **Fiber:** trace quantities (mostly from fruits, if used)

Cooking Tips:

- ❖ Experiment with different herb combinations until you find your favorites. Mint and cucumber, rosemary and grapefruit, and basil and strawberry are all fantastic matches.
- ❖ Be creative with fruits! Berries, citrus segments, apples, or even watermelon may lend a refreshing touch.
- ❖ To get a more powerful taste, slightly muddle the fruits and herbs before infusing.
- ❖ Repurpose your infused water by making salad dressings, marinades, or yogurt parfaits with any remaining fruits and herbs.

Health Benefits:

- ❖ Herbal infused water is a natural approach to enhance your water intake, which is necessary for good health.
- ❖ Different plants have various health advantages. Mint may help digestion and refresh breath, while rosemary helps improve memory and circulation.
- ❖ Fruits provide vitamins and antioxidants to your drink. Citrus fruits are exceptionally high in Vitamin C, which promotes immunity.
- ❖ Herbal infused water is a sugar-free and calorie-free method to flavor your water, making it an excellent choice for weight loss and healthy lifestyle.

3. Almond Butter and Banana Shake

- **Preparation time:** 5 minutes
- **Cooking time:** 0 minutes
- **Total time:** 5 minutes

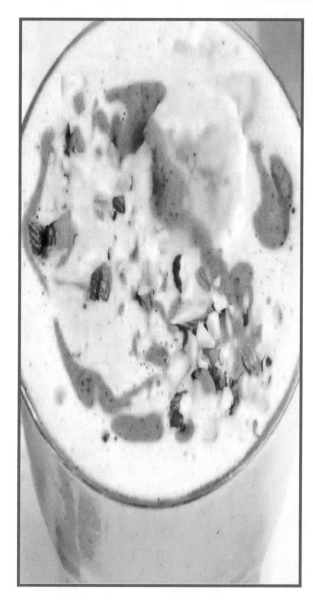

Ingredients:

- ❖ 1 cup unsweetened almond milk (or any milk of your choice)
- ❖ 1 medium frozen banana.
- ❖ 1/4 cup almond butter (creamy or crunchy, whatever you want)
- ❖ 1 teaspoon of vanilla extract (optional).
- ❖ 1/2 teaspoon of ground cinnamon (optional)
- ❖ A pinch of sea salt (optional).
- ❖ Use ice cubes as needed (if not using frozen bananas).

Instructions:

- ❖ Combine all items in a blender.
- ❖ Blend until smooth and creamy, adding additional almond milk or ice cubes as required to get the desired consistency.
- ❖ Enjoy right now!

This creamy and delicious almond butter and banana smoothie is an excellent healthy snack or breakfast choice. It's high in potassium, protein, and healthy fats, so you'll feel full and invigorated. Plus, it's very simple to create with only a few ingredients!

Serving size: Each recipe yields one serving.

Nutritional Information:

- ❖ **Calories:** around 300 (depending on the type of milk and nut butter used).
- ❖ **Carbohydrates:** 40 to 50 grams
- ❖ Fat: 10-15 g.
- ❖ **Protein:** 8–10 grams
- ❖ **Vitamin C:** 8% Daily Value (DV).
- ❖ **Potassium:** 15%. DV
- ❖ **Fiber:** 4-5 g

Cooking Tips:

- Use frozen bananas to make an extra-thick smoothie.
- If you don't have almond milk, you may use any other milk you choose.
- Add a scoop of protein powder to improve the protein content.
- Get creative with your add-ins! Spinach, berries, raw cacao powder, and a sprinkle of honey are all tasty possibilities.

Health Benefits:

- Bananas contain potassium, which is beneficial to heart health.
- Almond butter is a good source of protein and fat, which helps keep you full and content.
- This smoothie is also rich in vitamin C and fiber.

4. Herbal Teas to Relax

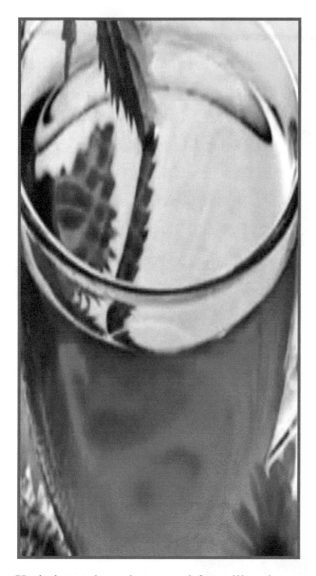

Herbal teas have been used for millennia to provide relaxation and stress relief. They are a natural method to unwind after a long day while also promoting emotions of serenity and quiet. This recipe provides a basic guidance for making your own soothing herbal tea mix, but feel free to experiment with other herbs to see what works best for you.

❖ **Preparation time:** 2 minutes

❖ **Cooking time:** 5 minutes

❖ **Total time:** 7 minutes

Ingredients:

❖ 1 cup water.

❖ 1 tablespoon dried herbs (chamomile, lavender, lemon balm, passionflower, or a mix)

❖ Honey or lemon (optional; to taste)

Instructions:

❖ Heat the water in a saucepan or teapot until it boils.

❖ Pour boiling water over dry herbs in a cup or infuser.

❖ Steep the tea for 5–10 minutes, depending on the desired strength.

❖ Strain the tea into a cup.

❖ If desired, season with honey or lemon juice.

Serving size per recipe: 1 mug.

Nutrition Information:

❖ **Calories:** 2 (without additional honey or lemon)

- ❖ **Carbohydrates:** 0.5 g (without additional honey or lemon)
- ❖ **Fat:** 0 g
- ❖ **Protein:** 0 grams.
- ❖ **Vitamin C** in trace levels (depending on the plants used)
- ❖ **Fiber:** trace quantities (dependent on the herbs used)

Cooking Tips:

- ❖ To make a stronger tea, use more dry herbs or simmer for a longer duration.
- ❖ You can experiment with different herb combinations to develop your own distinct flavor character.
- ❖ Dried fruits, such as rose hips or hibiscus, can be used to provide sweetness and vitamin C.
- ❖ Fresh herbs can also be utilized, however the amount will need to be adjusted according to their potency.

Health Benefits:

- ❖ Chamomile, lavender, lemon balm, and passionflower are all recognized for their soothing and relaxing effects.
- ❖ Herbal teas can also help you keep hydrated, which is essential for good health and well-being.
- ❖ Drinking warm drinks may also be pleasant and relaxing.

5. Green Tea and Blueberry Smoothie

❖ **Preparation time:** 5 minutes
❖ **Cooking Time:** 0 minutes
❖ **Total time:** 5 minutes

Ingredients:

❖ 1 cup of brewed green tea, cooled (see Cooking Tip for brewing directions).
❖ 1 cup of frozen blueberries.
❖ ½ frozen banana.
❖ 1/2 cup plain Greek yogurt.
❖ 1/4 cup unsweetened almond milk (or other plant-based milk).
❖ 1 tablespoon honey (optional)

Instructions:

❖ Combine all of the ingredients in a blender.
❖ Blend until smooth and creamy.
❖ Pour in a glass and enjoy!

Serving Size: 1 smoothie

Nutrition Information:

❖ **Calories:** 250–300 (depending on the ingredients)
❖ **Carbohydrates:** 40-50 grams
❖ **Fat:** 5-10g

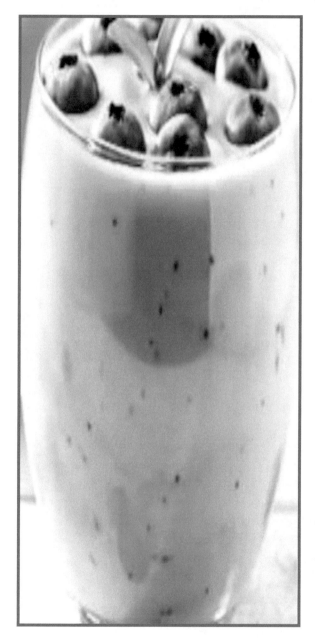

This refreshing smoothie is a tasty way to reap the health benefits of green tea and blueberries. It is high in antioxidants, vitamins, and minerals, making it ideal for breakfast or as a post-workout drink.

- ❖ **Protein:** 15-20 grams
- ❖ **Vitamin C:** An excellent source (from blueberries)
- ❖ **Fiber:** 5-7 grams

Cooking Tips:

- To make green tea, steep 1-2 bags in 1 cup of boiling water for 3-5 minutes. Remove the tea bags and allow the tea to cool fully before putting in the smoothie.
- Frozen bananas and blueberries make a thicker smoothie.
- Adjust the sweetness to your liking with honey or another natural sweetener.
- Add a scoop of protein powder to improve the protein content.

Health Benefits:

- ❖ Green tea has high levels of antioxidants, which can help protect your cells from harm.
- ❖ Blueberries are also abundant in antioxidants and have been linked to improved cognitive function.
- ❖ Greek yogurt contains protein and probiotics, which are beneficial to intestinal health.
- ❖ This smoothie has plenty of vitamins and minerals, including fiber and vitamin C.

6. Almond and Oat Milk Latte

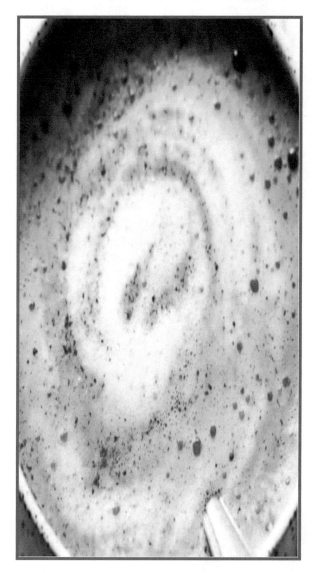

This Almond and Oat Milk Latte is a great dairy-free and lighter alternative to a conventional latte. It mixes the creamy smoothness of oat milk with the delicate nuttiness of almond milk, resulting in a delicious coffee drink. It's also high in nutrients and easy to modify to your liking.

❖ **Preparation time:** 5 minutes
❖ **Cooking time:** 2 minutes (depending on the heating technique)
❖ **Total time:** 7 minutes

Ingredients:

❖ 1 shot espresso (30 mL)
❖ 1/2 cup oat milk, unsweetened or vanilla-flavored
❖ 1/4 cup of unsweetened almond milk.
❖ 1/4 teaspoon of cinnamon (optional).
❖ To taste, add your preferred sweetener (honey, maple syrup, or sugar).

Instructions:

❖ Makc a new shot of espresso or use strong coffee.
❖ Warm the oat milk and almond milk in a small saucepan or heat-resistant cup over medium heat. Do not let it boil. Alternatively, use a milk frother to warm and froth the milk.
❖ If using, sprinkle cinnamon over the cup.
❖ Pour the espresso shot into a cup.

- Slowly pour the heated milk over the espresso, using a spoon to hold back the foam if desired.
- If used, adjust the sweetness to your liking.
- Gently whisk until combined, then top with a sprinkling of cinnamon or a dollop of froth if preferred.

Serving size: 1 latte.

Nutrition Facts: (approximate values per serving)

- **Calories:** 80–120 (depending on the sweetener used).
- **Carbohydrates:** 12-15 grams (depending on the sweetener chosen).
- **Fat:** 3-5g
- **Protein:** 2-3 grams.
- **Vitamin D:** enriched oat milk 20 IU
- **Fiber:** 1–2 grams

Cooking Tips:

- A double shot of espresso provides a fuller taste.
- If you don't have a milk frother, whisk the milk rapidly in a jug to make froth.

- Try out different tastes by adding a dash of vanilla extract, almond extract, or a touch of nutmeg.
- Heat the milk only until warm, not scorching. Overheating might change the flavor and texture.

Health Benefits:

- Dairy-free and vegan-friendly.
- Lower in calories and fat than a classic latte with full milk.
- Oat milk is a rich source of fiber and can aid digestion.
- Almond milk is an excellent source of vitamin E, an antioxidant.

7. Berries and Flaxseed Smoothie

- **Preparation time:** 5 minutes
- **Cooking time:** 0 minutes
- **Total time:** 5 minutes

Ingredients:

- ❖ 1-cup frozen mixed berries (strawberries, blueberries, raspberries)
- ❖ 1/2 cup fresh spinach.
- ❖ 1/2 cup plain, nonfat Greek yogurt.
- ❖ 1 tablespoon ground flaxseed.
- ❖ 1/2 cup unsweetened almond milk (or other milk of choice)
- ❖ 1/2 banana (optional)
- ❖ Add honey or maple syrup to taste.

Instructions:

- ❖ Combine all of the ingredients in a blender.
- ❖ Blend until smooth, scraping the sides as necessary.
- ❖ Add extra almond milk for a thinner smoothie, or a handful of ice cubes for a thicker one.
- ❖ If desired, add honey or maple syrup to taste and adjust for sweetness.

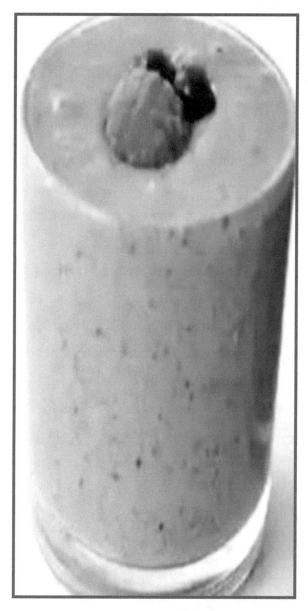

This tasty and nutritious Berry and Flaxseed Smoothie is an excellent way to begin the day or as a healthy and refreshing snack. This smoothie is high in antioxidants, fiber, and omega-3 fatty acids, so it will keep you pleased and energized.

Serving Size: 1 smoothie

Nutritional Information: (approximate value per serving)

- ❖ **Calories:** 250.
- ❖ **Carbohydrates:** 35 g
- ❖ **Fat:** 5g
- ❖ **Protein:** 10g
- ❖ **Vitamin C:** 40%. DV
- ❖ **Fiber:** 5 grams

Cooking Tips:

- ❖ Use frozen ripe bananas for a richer, creamier smoothie.
- ❖ If you don't have fresh spinach, you may use a handful of frozen spinach.
- ❖ Feel free to try different varieties of berries and milk.

- ❖ Add a scoop of protein powder to improve the protein content.

Health Benefits:

- ❖ Berries have high levels of antioxidants, which can help protect your cells from harm.
- ❖ Flaxseed is abundant in fiber and omega-3 fatty acids, which are beneficial to heart health and digestion.
- ❖ Spinach contains a variety of vitamins and minerals, including vitamin C, iron, and folate.
- ❖ Greek yogurt has protein, which can make you feel full and pleased.
- ❖ This smoothie is an excellent method to obtain a quick and simple boost of critical nutrients.

Chapter 10

Special Consideration

14-day MIND Diet Meal Plan

Day 1

Breakfast

Berry Blast Smoothie

Lunch

Spinach and Strawberry Salad

Snack

Almond and Walnut Mix

Dinner

Baked Salmon with Garlic and Herbs, Quinoa Pilaf with Herbs, and Steamed Asparagus with Lemon

Day 2

Breakfast

Oatmeal with Flax Seeds and Fresh Fruits

Lunch

Kale and Quinoa Salad with Lemon Dressing

Snack

Veggie Sticks with Hummus

Dinner

Turkey and Spinach Stuffed Peppers and Garlic Sautéed Spinach

Day 3

Breakfast

Nutty Banana Smoothie

Lunch

Mixed Greens with Berries and Nuts

Snack

Dark Chocolate and Walnut Bites

Dinner

Herb-Roasted Chicken with Vegetables and Roasted Brussels Sprouts with Almonds

Day 4

Breakfast

Greek Yogurt Parfait with Granola

Lunch

Lentil and Sweet Potato Curry

Snack

Apple Slices with Peanut Butter

Dinner

Grilled Shrimp with Quinoa Salad and Steamed Broccoli

Day 5

Breakfast

Quinoa Breakfast Bowl with Berries and Nuts

Lunch

Tuna and White Bean Salad

Snack

Roasted Chickpeas

Dinner

Stuffed Portobello Mushrooms and Brown Rice and Black Bean Salad

Day 6

Breakfast

Veggie-Packed Frittata

Lunch

Chickpea and Spinach Stew

Snack

Blueberry Almond Bars

Dinner

Lean Beef and Barley Stew and Steamed Carrots

Day 7

Breakfast

Whole Grain Avocado Toast

Lunch

Tomato Basil Soup with Whole Grain Croutons

Snack

Baked Apples with Cinnamon and Nuts

Dinner

Baked Salmon with Walnut Crust and Roasted Sweet Potatoes

Day 8

Breakfast

Berry and Oat Crisp

Lunch

Spinach and Strawberry Salad

Snack

Mixed Nuts

Dinner

Herb-Roasted Chicken with Vegetables and Steamed Green Beans

Day 9

Breakfast

Green Detox Smoothie

Lunch

Quinoa and Kale Salad

Snack

Dark Chocolate Avocado Mousse

Dinner

Lentil and Vegetable Soup and Roasted Brussels Sprouts

Day 10

Breakfast

Almond Butter and Banana Shake

Lunch

Spinach and Strawberry Salad

Snack

Pumpkin Seeds

Dinner

Turkey and Spinach Stuffed Peppers and Steamed Asparagus

Day 11

Breakfast

Greek Yogurt Parfait with Granola

Lunch

Mixed Greens with Berries and Nuts

Snack

Apple Slices with Peanut Butter

Dinner

Grilled Shrimp with Quinoa Salad and Steamed Broccoli

Day 12

Breakfast

Oatmeal with Flax Seeds and Fresh Fruits

Lunch

Tuna and White Bean Salad

Snack

Roasted Chickpeas

Dinner

Stuffed Portobello Mushrooms and Brown Rice and Black Bean Salad

Day 13

Breakfast

Veggie-Packed Frittata

Lunch

Chickpea and Spinach Stew

Snack

Blueberry Almond Bars

Dinner

Lean Beef and Barley Stew and Steamed Carrots

Day 14

Breakfast

Whole Grain Avocado Toast

Lunch

Tomato Basil Soup with Whole Grain Croutons

Snack

Baked Apples with Cinnamon and Nuts

Dinner

Baked Salmon with Walnut Crust and Roasted Sweet Potatoes

This meal plan provides a balanced and varied variety of MIND diet dishes, ensuring that you obtain the nutrients you need to maintain brain health while also eating great and fulfilling meals.

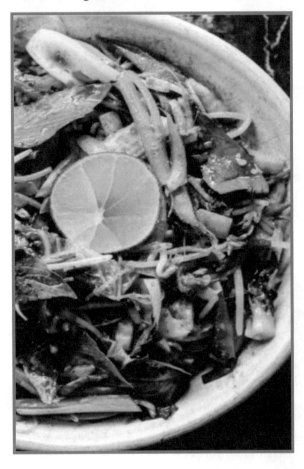

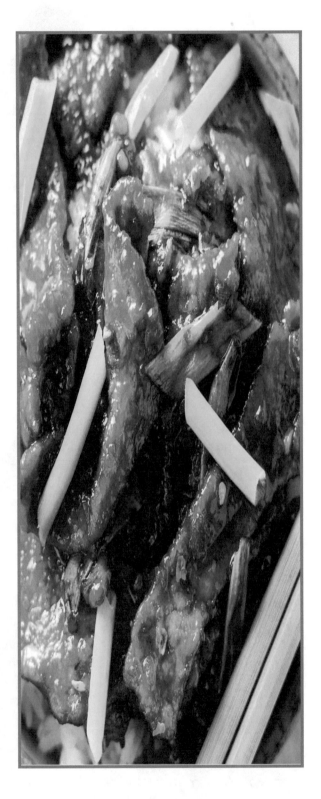

Making MIND Diet Choices at Restaurants

1. Research the Menu in Advance: Before going to a restaurant, look up the menu online. Look for recipes including MIND diet mainstays like leafy greens, seafood, nuts, and nutritious grains. Many restaurants provide their menus online, allowing you to make educated decisions ahead of time.

2. Go for Simple Preparations: Rather than frying, go for grilled, baked, steamed, or roasted foods. These cooking methods preserve the nutritional content of the food while reducing harmful fats.

3. Prioritize Vegetables: Start your dinner with a salad or a vegetable-based starter. Look for salads including lush greens, nuts, and a range of colorful veggies. To keep the quantity you consume under control, ask for dressings on the side.

4. Select Lean Proteins: Choose lean proteins such as fish, poultry, or lentils. Fish is a fantastic choice since it contains omega-3 fatty acids, which are good for brain function. Avoid breaded or fried meats in favor of grilled or baked options.

5. Request whole grains: Whenever feasible, choose for whole grains such as brown rice, quinoa, or whole wheat bread. If the menu does not list whole grain selections, ask your waitress.

6. Customize your order: Do not hesitate to request changes to make a dish healthy. For example, you can order more veggies, a side salad instead of fries, or sauces and dressings on the side.

7. Be Mindful of Portions: Restaurant servings are frequently bigger than required. Consider splitting a dish with a buddy or requesting a half-portion. You can also request a to-go box at the start of the meal and save half for later.

8. Stay hydrated: Drink water or unsweetened liquids with your meal. Avoid sugary beverages and restrict alcohol usage. If you decide to drink alcohol, a glass of red wine might be an excellent choice because it has potential brain health advantages when drunk in moderation.

9. Dessert Options: For dessert, choose fruit-based alternatives or split a modest serving with others. Fresh fruit, fruit sorbet, or a little piece of dark chocolate will satisfy your sweet need without throwing off your diet.

Quick and Healthy Options for Seniors on the Go

1. Pack your snacks: Prepare healthful snacks to take with you when out and about. Nuts, seeds, fresh fruit, and whole grain crackers are portable and healthy alternatives that are compatible with the MIND diet.

2. Choose Smart at Fast Food Restaurants: If you find yourself at a fast-food restaurant, choose healthier alternatives such as grilled chicken salads, whole grain wraps, or vegetable-based soups. Instead of fries and sugary drinks, choose water or an unsweetened beverage.

3. Visit grocery stores: Many grocery shops include salad bars, deli areas, and ready-to-eat meal alternatives. Choose from pre-cut veggies, fresh salads, grilled chicken, and whole grain salads. This can be a more convenient and nutritious alternative to typical fast food.

4. Search for Healthy Cafes: Look for cafes and eateries that promote fresh, healthy meals. Many restaurants now offer menu items that appeal to health-conscious customers, such as grain bowls, smoothie bowls, and avocado toast.

5. Stay prepared: Keep a supply of nutritious snacks in your car, purse, or bag. Nuts, dried fruit, and whole grain snacks may deliver a rapid energy boost without using harmful ingredients.

6. Go for Smoothies: Smoothie businesses may provide healthful and delicious meals on-the-go. Choose smoothies with greens, berries, nuts, and seeds, and avoid adding sweets or syrups.

7. Use Apps for Healthy Options: Use smartphone applications to identify healthy food alternatives in your area. Many applications include nutritional information and reviews, allowing you to make informed decisions fast.

8. Making Mindful Convenience Store Purchases: When visiting a convenience shop, search for nutritious snacks such as yogurt, fresh fruit, almonds, and whole grain crackers. Avoid sugary and processed meals.

9. Hydration On the Go: Carry a reusable water bottle with you to remain hydrated all day. Proper hydration is vital for general health and brain function.

10. Mindful eating: Take a minute to sit down and enjoy your food, even if you're on the run. Eating consciously allows you to savor your meal and realize when you're full, so reducing overeating.

By following these guidelines, you may enjoy dining out and discover quick, nutritious alternatives while sticking to the MIND diet. Making mindful decisions keeps you on track with your nutritional objectives and promotes general brain health, even when life becomes hectic.

Dietary Restrictions and Allergies

Adapting the MIND diet to meet dietary limitations and allergies is critical to ensuring that everyone benefits from its brain-boosting effects. The MIND diet may be modified to match your unique goals, such as avoiding gluten and dairy or managing certain health disorders like diabetes or weight concerns.

Gluten-free MIND Diet Recipes

Individuals with gluten sensitivity or celiac disease must completely eliminate gluten from their diets. Fortunately, many MIND diet foods are inherently gluten-free.

Gluten-free grains:

- ❖ Quinoa may be used in salads, as a side dish, or to make breakfast porridge.
- ❖ Brown rice is a versatile grain that may be cooked in soups, stews, and stir-fries.
- ❖ Millet: Another gluten-free grain that works great as a salad or side dish.
- ❖ Oats (certified gluten-free) are great for porridge, smoothies, and baking.

Dairy-free Options

For people who are lactose intolerant or allergic to dairy, there are several dairy-free options that follow the MIND diet principles.

Dairy-free Alternatives:

- ❖ Almond Milk: Add almond milk to smoothies, porridge, and baking.

- ❖ Coconut Yogurt is a dairy-free choice for parfaits, smoothies, and snacks.
- ❖ Nutritional yeast provides a cheese taste without dairy, making it ideal for flavoring veggies and popcorn.

Adapting the Mind Diet

For diabetic seniors:

Controlling blood sugar levels is critical for diabetic elders.

The MIND diet may be tailored to fit the demands of diabetics by emphasizing foods with a low glycemic index and monitoring carbohydrate intake.

Tips:

- ❖ **Prioritize Whole Grains:** To help control blood sugar, choose whole grains such as quinoa, brown rice, and oats over processed grains.
- ❖ **Increase Fiber Intake:** To assist regulate blood sugar levels, eat lots of veggies, legumes, and nuts.
- ❖ **Healthy Fats:** Consume healthy fats from avocados, nuts, seeds, and olive oil.

For weight management:

If you want to lose weight while also improving your mental health, the MIND diet can help you do it.

Tips:

- ❖ **Portion Control:** Be cautious of portion sizes to avoid overeating, especially when eating calorie-dense foods such as nuts and seeds.
- ❖ **Balanced Meals:** To keep you full and happy, make sure each meal has a good balance of protein, healthy fats, and fiber-rich veggies.
- ❖ **Limit Added Sugars:** Avoid meals and beverages with added sugars and instead consume naturally sweet foods such as fruits in moderation.

Making these changes, you may adjust the MIND diet to different dietary constraints and health circumstances, ensuring that it remains an effective tool for sustaining cognitive performance and general well-being. Whether you need to avoid gluten and dairy, manage diabetes, or lose weight, the MIND diet has adaptable and healthy options to match your goals.

CONCLUSION

The MIND diet is more than simply a method of eating; it's a holistic strategy for preserving and improving brain function as we age. The MIND diet enhances general well-being and reduces the risk of cognitive decline by emphasizing nutrient-dense meals that support cognitive function. Incorporating a mix of fruits, vegetables, whole grains, nuts, seafood, and healthy fats into your daily diet will improve your mental clarity, memory, and general well-being.

Perfect Tips for Following MIND Diet Recipes

1. Start gradually: Begin by applying MIND diet ideas to your existing eating patterns. Replace less healthful options with nutrient-dense alternatives, such as replacing refined grains with whole grains or snacking on nuts and seeds rather than processed meals.

2. Plan your weekly meals and snacks: This ensures that you have the right components on hand and may make better choices. Use a variety of recipes to make your dinners interesting and pleasurable.

3. Stay informed: Learn about brain-healthy foods. Understanding the "why" behind the MIND diet will help you stick to it. Understanding the individual advantages of certain meals can also help you make smarter decisions.

4. Experiment with different recipes and cooking techniques: Experimenting with new products and flavors may help keep your meals interesting and prevent diet burnout.

5. To stay on track with the MIND diet, prepare ingredients and meals ahead of time. Batch preparing and portioning meals can help you save time and avoid the temptation to choose less healthful choices.

6. Aim for balance and moderation in your meals, including a range of food categories. Moderation is crucial, so indulge on your favorite foods periodically without feeling bad.

7. Stay Hydrated: Drink lots of water all day. Proper hydration is vital for general health and brain function.

8. Maintain an active lifestyle by including regular physical exercise into your diet. Exercise promotes brain health and well-being. Choose activities that you love, such as walking, yoga, or dancing.

9. Get support by sharing your story with family and friends. Having a support system may keep you motivated and accountable. Consider joining a club or finding a diet buddy to swap recipes and suggestions.

10. Pay attention to your body's response to different meals. Everyone's body responds differently, so tailor your diet to your specific health and wellness objectives.

Following these suggestions and embracing the MIND diet concepts, you may take proactive measures toward preserving cognitive health and living a bright, full life. The road to greater brain health is gratifying, with tasty meals and the satisfaction of knowing you're nurturing your mind and body for the future. The MIND diet can help you become healthier, smarter, and more energetic!

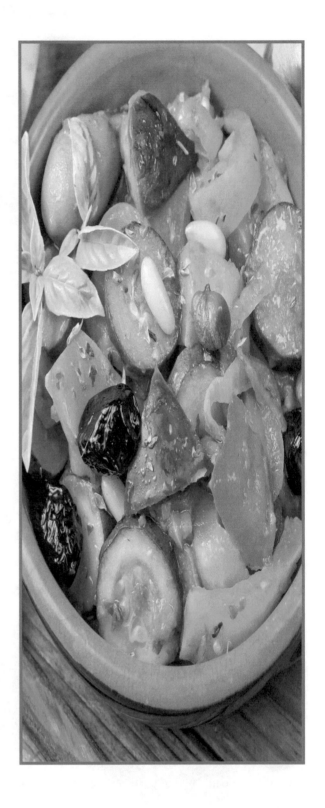

Bonus Section

Bonus 1: Email Of Consultation

Dear valued reader,

Thank you for selecting **"MIND Diet Cookbook for Seniors 2024."** Your commitment to invest in your health and well-being is admirable, and I hope this cookbook has been a helpful resource on your path to greater brain health.

Your feedback is extremely important to us, and we would be grateful if you could take the time to post a favorable review. Let us know what you liked best about the book, whether it was the diversity of recipes, the meal planning, the helpful hints, or anything else that stuck out to you.

As a mark of our thanks, we are providing one additional consultation by email. If you have any questions or concerns concerning the book, please contact us at **hmillerelva@gmail.com**. I will gladly assist and support you.

Thank you for your continued support and for being a member of our community. Your positive rating and feedback allow us to continue providing useful tools for others on their cooking journeys.

Bonus 2: Effective Exercises to Help You Stay Healthy

Scan Here

To claim these bonuses with ease, kindly scan the Q.R Code above.

Thanks!!!

Meal

Planner Journal

Meal Planner Journal

Monday

Breakfast | Lunch | Dinner

Tuesday

Breakfast | Lunch | Dinner

Wednesday

Breakfast | Lunch | Dinner

Thursday

Breakfast | Lunch | Dinner

Friday

Breakfast | Lunch | Dinner

SaturdAY/sUNDAY

Breakfast

Lunch

Dinner

Note

Meal Planner Journal

Monday

Breakfast	Lunch	Dinner

Tuesday

Breakfast	Lunch	Dinner

Wednesday

Breakfast	Lunch	Dinner

Thursday

Breakfast	Lunch	Dinner

Friday

Breakfast	Lunch	Dinner

SaturdAY/sUNDAY

Breakfast

Lunch

Dinner

Note

Meal Planner Journal

Monday

Breakfast	Lunch	Dinner

Tuesday

Breakfast	Lunch	Dinner

Wednesday

Breakfast	Lunch	Dinner

Thursday

Breakfast	Lunch	Dinner

Friday

Breakfast	Lunch	Dinner

SaturdAY/sUNDAY

Breakfast
_____

Lunch
_____

Dinner
_____

Note

Meal Planner Journal

Monday

Breakfast	Lunch	Dinner

Tuesday

Breakfast	Lunch	Dinner

Wednesday

Breakfast	Lunch	Dinner

Thursday

Breakfast	Lunch	Dinner

Friday

Breakfast	Lunch	Dinner

SaturdAY/SUNDAY

Breakfast
_____

Lunch
_____

Dinner
_____

Note

Meal Planner Journal

Monday

Breakfast	Lunch	Dinner

Tuesday

Breakfast	Lunch	Dinner

Wednesday

Breakfast	Lunch	Dinner

Thursday

Breakfast	Lunch	Dinner

Friday

Breakfast	Lunch	Dinner

SaturdAY/sUNDAY

Breakfast

Lunch

Dinner

Note

Meal Planner Journal

Monday
Breakfast	Lunch	Dinner

Tuesday
Breakfast	Lunch	Dinner

Wednesday
Breakfast	Lunch	Dinner

Thursday
Breakfast	Lunch	Dinner

Friday
Breakfast	Lunch	Dinner

SaturdAY/SUNDAY

Breakfast

Lunch

Dinner

Note

Meal Planner Journal

Monday

Breakfast	Lunch	Dinner

Tuesday

Breakfast	Lunch	Dinner

Wednesday

Breakfast	Lunch	Dinner

Thursday

Breakfast	Lunch	Dinner

Friday

Breakfast	Lunch	Dinner

SaturdAY/SUNDAY

Breakfast

Lunch

Dinner

Note

Meal Planner Journal

Monday

Breakfast	Lunch	Dinner

Tuesday

Breakfast	Lunch	Dinner

Wednesday

Breakfast	Lunch	Dinner

Thursday

Breakfast	Lunch	Dinner

Friday

Breakfast	Lunch	Dinner

SaturdAY/SUNDAY

Breakfast

Lunch

Dinner

Note

Meal Planner Journal

Monday

Breakfast	Lunch	Dinner

Tuesday

Breakfast	Lunch	Dinner

Wednesday

Breakfast	Lunch	Dinner

Thursday

Breakfast	Lunch	Dinner

Friday

Breakfast	Lunch	Dinner

SaturdAY/sUNDAY

Breakfast

Lunch

Dinner

Note

Meal Planner Journal

Monday

Breakfast	Lunch	Dinner

Tuesday

Breakfast	Lunch	Dinner

Wednesday

Breakfast	Lunch	Dinner

Thursday

Breakfast	Lunch	Dinner

Friday

Breakfast	Lunch	Dinner

SaturdAY/sUNDAY

Breakfast

Lunch

Dinner

Note

Made in United States
Troutdale, OR
09/27/2024